Workplace-Based Assessments in Psychiatric Training

Workplace-Based Assessments in Psychiatric Training

Edited by

Dinesh Bhugra

Amit Malik

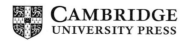

CAMBRIDGE
UNIVERSITY PRESS

CAMBRIDGE UNIVERSITY PRESS
Cambridge, New York, Melbourne, Madrid, Cape Town,
Singapore, São Paulo, Delhi, Tokyo, Mexico City

Cambridge University Press
The Edinburgh Building, Cambridge CB2 8RU, UK

Published in the United States of America by Cambridge University Press, New York

www.cambridge.org
Information on this title: www.cambridge.org/9780521131803

First published 2011

Printed in the United Kingdom at the University Press, Cambridge

A catalogue record for this publication is available from the British Library

ISBN 978-0-521-13180-3 Paperback

This book is dedicated to Satya and Prabhu Dayal Goswami, for their love, support and blessings

Contents

Contributors

Joan Anzia
Residency Training Director
Associate Professor of Psychiatry
Department of Psychiatry and Behavioural Sciences
Feinberg School of Medicine
Northwestern Memorial Hospital
Chicago, IL
USA

Dinesh Bhugra
Professor of Mental Health and Cultural Diversity
Health Service and Population Research Department
Institute of Psychiatry
King's College London
UK

Philip Boyce
Professor of Psychiatry
Sydney Medical School
University of Sydney, and
Head of the Perinatal Psychiatry Service
Westmead Hospital
Australia

Andrew Brittlebank
The Fairnington Centre
Hexham
Northumberland
UK

Prabha S. Chandra
Professor of Psychiatry

National Institute of Mental Health and Neurosciences
Bangalore
India

Santosh K. Chaturvedi
Professor and Head, Department of Psychiatry
National Institute of Mental Health and Neurosciences
Bangalore
India

Jim Crossley
Consultant Paediatrician and Senior Research Fellow
Academic Unit of Medical Education
University of Sheffield
Sheffield
UK

Mark Davies
Education Project Officer
The Royal Australian and New Zealand College of Psychiatrists
Victoria
Australia

Amit Malik
Clinical Services Director and Consultant Psychiatrist
Hampshire Partnership NHS Foundation Trust
Gosport
Hampshire
UK

John Manring
Associate Professor
Psychiatry and Behavioural Sciences
Upstate Medical University
Syracuse, NY
USA

Charlotte Ringsted
Professor of Medical Education
Director of Centre for Clinical Education
University of Copenhagen and The Capital Region
Rigshospitalet
Denmark

Karen Saperson
Associate Professor and Head
Division of Geriatric Psychiatry
Department of Psychiatry and Behavioural Neurosciences

McMaster University
Hamilton, ONT
Canada

Christine Spratt
Education and Curriculum Advisor
The Royal Australian and New Zealand College of Psychiatrists
Victoria
Australia

Richard Summers
Clinical Associate Professor of Psychiatry
Co-Director of Residency Training
Department of Psychiatry
University of Pennsylvania
Philadelphia, PA
USA

Richard P. Swinson
Professor Emeritus
Department of Psychiatry and Behavioural Neurosciences
Michael G de Groote School of Medicine
McMaster University
Hamilton, ON
Canada

Jagadisha Thirthalli
Associate Professor of Psychiatry
National Institute of Mental Health and Neurosciences
Bangalore
India

Valerie Wass
Professor of Medical Education
Head of School of Medicine
Keele University
Staffordshire
UK

Priyanthy Weerasekera
Associate Professor
Postgraduate Psychotherapy Coordinator
Department of Psychiatry and Behavioural Neurosciences
McMaster University
Hamilton, ONT
Canada

Preface

The Royal College of Psychiatrists began exploring the issue of implementing workplace-based assessments in psychiatric training in the UK in 2005. Initial scoping of the assessment methods in other countries and then a formal literature review made us realize the paucity of international literature on how psychiatric trainees are assessed in training systems around the globe. After painstaking investigation, it became clear that most national and regional postgraduate assessment programmes were still using traditional knowledge-based assessments to evaluate their trainees and certify them for independent practice. The difficulties in obtaining this information actually prompted the idea of having one resource specific to psychiatry that would outline developments in postgraduate psychiatric assessments internationally and place them within the context of the current evidence base in evaluating trainee or resident performance.

This volume will outline the current evidence base in assessing postgraduate trainees, especially in the context of their workplace. The specific research messages regarding different types of workplace-based assessment methodologies will also be reviewed. Subsequent chapters will look at assessment practices in a range of postgraduate psychiatric training systems across the globe, with a special emphasis on workplace-based or in-training assessments. Some of these are national systems, whilst others exist within a postgraduate psychiatric training institution and have been selected for their innovation and initiative within a national or international context. Methods and issues relating to the assessment of the patients' perspective of a trainee's performance will be discussed. Finally, we will aim to look to the future and the various challenges facing workplace-based assessments in postgraduate psychiatric training, focusing especially on some of the challenges arising from the principles outlined in the introductory chapter.

We are grateful to all the psychiatric and medical educators who have contributed to this book. Their leadership and contributions in the area of assessing postgraduate trainees have led to significant improvements in this field internationally and added to the richness of this text. As always, we remain grateful to our respective departments, both at the Institute of Psychiatry at King's College

London and the Hampshire Partnership NHS Foundation Trust, who support us in our endeavours in improving postgraduate psychiatric education. The Royal College of Psychiatrists has always been a champion of innovation in psychiatric education and our involvement in its activities is the basis for all our work in this area. Thanks also go to Richard Marley and his colleagues at CUP for their support and encouragement. Finally, this volume could not have been accomplished without the painstaking efforts of Andrea Livingstone, who has the unique ability to bring together pieces of written work and make them gel together into a readable textbook.

Dinesh Bhugra and Amit Malik

Workplace-based assessments in psychiatry: setting the scene

Amit Malik and Dinesh Bhugra

Background: changing socio-political context

Over the last decade the socio-political world within which medicine exists has changed significantly. The expectations of medicine as a profession, and doctors as its constituent members, have morphed drastically and the role of the physician has transformed from an autocratic decision-maker to a collaborative facilitator for patients in supporting them to make complex healthcare decisions. National and international high-profile healthcare scandals have also meant that governments, and through them the public, now expect greater transparency in the standards to which doctors are trained and demand evidence that trained doctors have actually met these standards before they are allowed into independent practice. Additionally, there are public and professional expectations that fully trained doctors are evaluated at regular intervals to ensure that they are up to date with the latest developments and have maintained the professional skills that enable them to practise medicine.

Moreover, all this is happening when, on the one hand, quite appropriately, an emphasis on patient safety has necessitated a reduction in the working hours of trainees around the world and, on the other hand, many healthcare training systems are being encouraged to shorten the length of training, to meet healthcare workforce needs and to reduce the overall cost of training. Therefore, one can no longer rely on the traditional apprenticeship model where trainees were expected to spend long hours over a number of years in training with the hope that they would have enough experience and would have learnt sufficiently by osmosis to enable them to practise independently. Instead, training has had to become more structured, efficient and outcome-orientated, to ensure that trainees engage in educationally valuable activities to attain competencies that have been defined in a curriculum that is 'fit for the purpose' to prepare the needs of their professional

Workplace-Based Assessments in Psychiatric Training, ed. Dinesh Bhugra and Amit Malik.
Published by Cambridge University Press. © Cambridge University Press 2011.

practice on completion of training. Additionally, trainees must undergo assessment to demonstrate that they have attained these competencies.

However, socio-political factors are not the only reason for changes in the world of postgraduate medical education. For decades, assessments in medical training have relied on the evaluation of a postgraduate trainee's knowledge or skills in one-off high-stake encounters rather than focusing on their ability to acquire competencies and perform in the workplace. This has created perverse incentives for learning amongst postgraduate medical trainees and fostered a medical education system that, some would argue, has created 'competent' doctors despite of rather than because of it.

This introductory chapter discusses some of the rationale for the changes in postgraduate medical assessments, including the introduction and implementation of workplace-based assessments as components of assessment systems. It also outlines the formative and summative role of all assessments and contextualizes assessments within educational programmes based on competency-based curricula. Finally, it introduces some of the technical and psychometric considerations that must be taken into account when developing assessment systems for postgraduate medical training.

Rationale for workplace-based assessment

For decades, postgraduate medical assessments have focused on assessing knowledge in one-off high-stake examinations. Since the 1980s, in addition to assessments of knowledge, these examinations have progressed to include skills assessments, such as the long case examination and objective structured clinical examinations (OSCEs). However, as Miller outlined in his landmark discourse in 1990, clinical competencies need to be assessed at four different levels, which he draws on a pyramid: 'knows', 'knows how', 'shows how' and 'does'. Workplace-based assessments (WPBAs) target 'does' – the highest level of Miller's pyramid, as this involves assessing a trainee's actual performance in the workplace (Miller, 1990). It is particularly important to assess performance in the workplace throughout the duration of training, for a variety of reasons.

Firstly, workplace-based assessments allow for a more authentic evaluation of how a trainee would respond in a real-life situation compared with the artificial circumstances of an examination. Secondly, assessing trainees on a regular basis within the context of the workplace provides greater opportunities for diagnosing developmental needs at an early stage and delivering regular formative feedback throughout training rather than at a few discrete points in high-stake situations. Thirdly, having a number of assessments over the training period allows for greater sampling of the curriculum than would be feasible in periodic examinations. In addition, having assessments from a number of assessors enables a greater triangulation of information to assess a trainee's competence and mitigates some of the concerns around inter-rater reliability in examination settings with a limited number of assessors assessing over a short period of time. Finally, it is now clear that assessments drive learning and that assessing trainees for their performance in all professional domains (clinical and non-clinical) in real-life situations will enable them to develop such professional skills as teamworking, forming relationships with colleagues and leadership, which are often not easily tested in artificial examination contexts.

All this is not to say that workplace-based assessments are superior to examinations, as examinations provide a degree of externality and standardization that plays a crucial role in providing confidence in the very high-stake decisions that allow a medical trainee to undertake independent clinical practice with patients. The above rationale merely supports a case for developing an assessment programme that includes both workplace-based assessments and external examinations, where the overall high-stake pass–fail decisions are made by taking evidence from both these sources in addition to the professional judgement of experienced educational and clinical supervisors in the workplace.

Purpose of workplace-based assessments

To engender stakeholder trust within an assessment programme, the purpose of its various component assessments should be explicit from the outset. The two main purposes of assessment are *for learning* (formative) and *of learning* (summative) (Wass *et al.*, 2001). This distinction, however, is a lot more artificial and complex in actual practice: some of the evidence from formative assessments, such as workplace-based assessments, is often used for making summative decisions, and the feedback from summative assessments, such as examinations, can often clarify developmental needs. Rather than attempting to create an artificial and impossible distinction between formative and summative assessments, assessment programme developers should ensure that the different purposes of assessments are clarified to examiners from the outset and all efforts are made to ensure that individual assessments are psychometrically, logistically and educationally fit for their intended purposes.

Curriculum development and blueprinting

Whilst it is beyond the scope of this book to discuss the principles and process of curriculum development, suffice it to say that outcome-based curricula must be developed to define the competencies that a fully trained medical professional must possess in a particular specialty at a particular time. Assessment systems must be embedded within these outcome-based curricula and must consist of a range of assessments that assess the various domains of the curriculum.

Two principles should be taken into account whilst doing this. Firstly, the test content should be planned in relation to the learning outcomes by the process of blueprinting. A blueprint is a matrix in which the test designer decides how many items/tasks are to be assessed for each subject or category (Holsgrove *et al.*, 2009). Secondly, the blueprinting should also ensure that the format of an assessment is appropriate for the domain (such as knowledge, skills or attitudes) of the curriculum that it intends to assess (Wass *et al.*, 2001). Both these steps are crucial to ensure the validity of individual assessments and the overall assessment system.

Utility of assessments

In his seminal paper, Cees van der Vleuten (1996) defined the concept of utility as a multiplicative product of reliability, validity, educational impact, acceptability and cost. Describing perfect utility as a utopia, he used the model to describe the compromises and trade-offs between the constituent variables of utility, depending on the context and purpose of the assessment. In designing assessment tools and programmes, each of these variables must be considered and it would be prudent to discuss them in a bit more detail here.

Reliability

Reliability is a measure of how reproducible and consistent a test's results are (Wass *et al.*, 2001). Many factors influence the overall reliability of an assessment, including assessor factors, clinical case and the context of the assessment. Cronbach's α (alpha) is a well-recognized contemporary measure of internal consistency used by test developers. Its value ranges from 0 to 1; the requisite value for a particular assessment depends on the purpose of the assessment. As a general principle, the higher the stakes, the greater the value of α that is required for an assessment. For instance, whilst $\alpha \geq 0.9$ would be desirable in high-stake examinations, $\alpha \leq 0.8$ might be acceptable for workplace-based assessment (Holsgrove *et al.*, 2009).

Different assessors rate trainees differently for similar performances and some of this error can be minimized by assessor training and standardization of rating scales. However, to ensure greater inter-rater reliability of workplace-based assessments, several assessors should be used to triangulate the assessment information across a range of contexts. It is now also known that trainees perform differently across clinical cases and that, notwithstanding generic skills such as communication, performance measurement is task-specific and doctors perform differently at different tasks. Therefore, there should be adequate sampling from the curriculum to assess trainees across a range of clinical cases (van der Vleuten, 1996).

However, it has recently been argued that it is not sufficient merely to regard assessors as *interchangeable measurement instruments*, whereby lack of reliability or consistency can be resolved simply by enhancing the standardization and objectivity of assessment tools or increasing inter-rater reliability by assessor training. Such a great reliance solely on a psychometric approach might ignore the influence of assessors' personal and organizational perspectives on the overall performance measurement, as well as the *clinical, organizational and social context* within which the assessment takes place, especially in workplace-based assessments. Assessors must be seen as actively making complex professional judgements and it must be recognized that contextual factors have a significant influence on this process. It is very important to understand the assessors' judgement and decision-making processes from a social-cognitive perspective and the environmental factors that affect assessors' motivation and goals (Govaerts *et al.*, 2007)

Validity

Validity is a measure of how thoroughly a test assesses what it purports to assess. Messick (1995) defines validity as:

The degree to which empirical evidence and theoretical rationales support the adequacy and appropriateness of inferences and actions based on test scores or other models of assessment.

Traditionally, validity has been classified into three types – content, construct and criterion, where criterion validity is further divided into predictive and concurrent validity. There have been criticisms of the concept of face validity (does a test appear to assess what it claims to?) (Streiner and Norman, 2003). A more contemporary view also sees all validity as being construct validity. The current state-of-the-art view is that validity is a process of hypothesis testing, wherein the aim of a validation study is to formulate a hypothesis about the inferences that can be drawn from the results of an assessment and then to collect evidence to prove or disprove the hypothesis (Downing and Haladyna, 2004).

Appropriate blueprinting of assessments of a curriculum supports the content validity of the assessment framework. Concurrent validity models (e.g., workplace-based assessment with national written examinations) must be evaluated, especially where the same curriculum domains are being assessed.

Predictive validity studies using longitudinal data (e.g., success in workplace-based assessments predicting clinical or examination success) are important in enhancing the validity and acceptability of assessment programmes. Qualitative evaluation methods (such as surveys and focus groups) can be used to assess the consequential validity (e.g., educational impact) of workplace-based assessment (Holsgrove *et al.*, 2009).

Educational impact

Assessments strongly influence learning in a variety of ways and therefore have a significant educational impact (Wass *et al.*, 2001). The content, format, feedback and scheduling of assessments all influence what and how trainees learn from the curriculum (van der Vleuten, 1996). The challenge, therefore, for developers of assessments and assessment systems is to utilize this knowledge in developing assessment systems that promote the curriculum objectives and outcomes.

Especially in busy vocational learning environments, such as postgraduate medical training, trainees will always prioritize learning components of the curriculum that are assessed most frequently, or most thoroughly, or to which greatest importance is attached within the overall programme outcome (van der Vleuten, 1996). Therefore, whilst blueprinting is important to ensure adequate sampling of the curriculum, it is also crucial to ensure that trainees learn the most important components of the curriculum most effectively. The content of the assessment programme should give consistent messages regarding this.

Ideally, a variety of assessment formats should be used within an assessment system with each format validated for a particular purpose. Additionally, the same format can be used to assess different aspects of the curriculum (Holsgrove et al., 2009). It is important to recognize the intended and unintended consequences of assessment formats, and their evaluation and ongoing analysis are crucial in managing and responding to these consequences when they occur (van der Vleuten, 1996).

Feedback must constitute an indispensable part of assessments and assessment programmes as it contributes significantly to the educational impact of assessments and the trainee's learning experience. It is postulated that in the context of postgraduate medical training, facilitative rather than directive feedback is more effective. Feedback should relate to tasks, be specific instead of general and relate to the individual (Archer, 2010). To achieve this, workplace-based assessments should be viewed as structured and regular feedback opportunities and feedback given should link to action planning and the trainee's overall learning plan. All this can only be attained if a culture of reflection is developed within training healthcare organizations and trainers are trained to facilitate effective, formative and action-orientated feedback (Holsgrove et al., 2009).

Finally, the frequency, timing and relation to progression have a huge effect on the educational impact of assessments, and careful and conscious consideration should be given to these factors by the designers of assessment programmes (van der Vleuten, 1996).

Acceptability

Assessment tools and programmes that do not enjoy stakeholder acceptability, especially from trainees and assessors, will not succeed. Dijkstra et al. (2010) outline the prerequisites for trust in and acceptability of assessment systems previously detailed in the literature. These include authenticity, fairness, honesty, transparency of procedures (due process), well-defined roles and high-quality feedback (Govaerts et al., 2007). Additionally, including assessors in the development of assessment tools and programmes enhances the acceptability of the assessment tools and programmes. It is also important that there is clear communication between the programme developers and the assessors and trainees regarding the outcome measures set out within the curriculum, their relative significance and their correspondence to the domains on the assessment tools.

A clear, unambiguous and explicit message needs to be relayed to assessors and trainees regarding the purpose of assessments and the manner in which assessment results will be used. All stakeholders must be actively encouraged to provide feedback on the assessment programme and this should be utilized to make positive modifications to the programme. Finally, employing organizations must provide support for assessments to be carried out not only by ensuring that time and other resources are made available – an area that will be covered next when considering the issue of cost – but also by promoting an organizational culture that values honest feedback and reflection in order to promote the development of competent and reflective specialists (Govaerts *et al.*, 2007).

Cost

There are significant overt costs involved in developing, delivering and evaluating assessment methods and programmes. It is important, right at the outset of assessment programme development, to address this issue in two ways. Firstly, the assessment programme developers must identify the funding resources for the various stages of assessment development and delivery and, secondly, they must explore innovative ways in which these costs can be minimized, for example by using information technology systems rather than paper assessments and by sharing assessment delivery at a regional or national level. For instance, in the UK, workplace-based assessments are delivered across all training programmes using a national IT system.

However, there are significant covert costs involved, especially in the delivery of assessment systems, including assessor and trainee time to undertake assessments and provide or receive regular feedback. As already stated, it is crucial that employing organizations make time and resources available to assessors and trainees to ensure that detailed and valid assessments can take place and structured feedback can be provided to trainees.

Assessments as components of educational programmes

The medical education literature is flooded with evaluations of different workplace-based assessment tools. However, concerns have been raised in more recent work, regarding the relative absence of a systematic approach to assessments. This involves having a clear set of outcomes (or competencies) that are expected of a postgraduate medical training programme. Various assessment methods and their content should then be clearly specified, to ensure that there is adequate sampling across all outcomes (blueprinting) and appropriate assessment formats are utilized for assessing different competencies. Addressing assessments in this way will also help in reducing the overlap between the areas assessed by different assessments; allowing weaknesses of some assessments to be compensated by strengths of others and assisting in the triangulation of information from a range of sources, especially whilst making high-stake decisions (Dijkstra *et al.*, 2010).

Conclusion

This chapter has aimed to set the context for the assessment of trainee performance in the workplace during postgraduate psychiatric training. A clear message is that developing and delivering a successful assessment programme is not only a psychometric issue but is also a cultural, political and economic one. There is an overall note of caution in overemphasizing the psychometric principles at the expense of educational and social-cognitive ones. Moreover, the responsibility lies with us, the psychiatric profession, to ensure that we set out clear outcomes for our trainees within training programmes and then ensure that these outcomes are adequately assessed by an assessment programme. This is crucial not only to develop 'fit-for-the-purpose' psychiatrists for tomorrow but also to ensure that we protect our patients and maintain wider public confidence and trust within the psychiatric profession.

REFERENCES

Archer, J. C. (2010). State of the science in health professional education: effective feedback. *Medical Education*, **44**, 101–108.

Dijkstra, J., van der Vleuten, C. P. M. and Schuwirth, L. W. T. (2010). A new framework for designing programmes of assessment. *Advances in Health Sciences Education*, **15**(3), 379–393.

Downing, S. M. and Haladyna, T. M. (2004). Validity threats: overcoming interference with proposed interpretations of assessment data. *Medical Education*, **38**, 327–333.

Govaerts, M. J. B., van der Vleuten, C. P. M., Schuwirth, L. W. T. and Muijtjens, A. M. M. (2007). Broadening perspectives on clinical performance assessment: rethinking the nature of in-training assessment. *Advances in Health Sciences Education*, **12**, 239–260.

Holsgrove, G., Malik, A. and Bhugra, D. (2009). The postgraduate curriculum and assessment programme in psychiatry: the underlying principles. *Advances in Psychiatric Treatment*, **15**, 114–122.

Messick, S. (1995). Standards of validity and the validity of standards in performance assessment. *Educational Measurement: Issues and Practice*, **14**, 5–8.

Miller, G. E. (1990). The assessment of clinical skills/competence/performance. *Academic Medicine*, **65**(9), S63–S67.

Streiner, D. L. and Norman, G. R. (2003). *Health Measurement Scales: A Practical Guide to Their Development and Use*, 3rd edn. Oxford: Oxford University Press.

van der Vleuten, C. P. M. (1996). The assessment of professional competence: developments, research and practical implications. *Advances in Health Sciences Education*, **1**, 41–67.

Wass, V., van der Vleuten, C., Shatzer, J. and Jones, R. (2001). Assessment of clinical competence. *The Lancet*, **357**, 945–949.

2

Workplace-based assessments – an evidence-based overview

Amit Malik and Dinesh Bhugra

Editors' introduction

In many parts of the world, workplace-based assessment methods now constitute an indispensable component of assessment systems in postgraduate psychiatric training. The previous chapter outlined the theoretical background for workplace-based assessments, including some of the technical considerations of their development, implementation and evaluation. This chapter aims to classify different methods by which postgraduate medical trainees can be assessed in the workplace, and a brief discussion follows of the contemporary evidence related to some of these assessment methods. It is inevitable that some assessments work better than others, and the supporting literature varies depending upon how long a tool has been used and how its validity is assessed. Both assessors and trainees need to be aware of the pros and cons of the various assessments and use them accordingly.

Classification of workplace-based assessments

Various workplace-based tools are being used and different aspects of their utility have been analyzed. It is crucial that assessment methods are developed and used as part of a pragmatic approach rather than as individual assessment tools that do not relate to each other as components of the relevant curriculum. Careful consideration also needs to be given to the content and format of assessments to ensure that they sample the curriculum efficiently and effectively and validly assess the intended aspects of a trainee's competencies.

Reviewing the literature (C. Fitch, A. Malik and P. Lelliott, personal communication, 2009), it is possible to classify the assessment tools into three distinct categories:

Workplace-Based Assessments in Psychiatric Training, ed. Dinesh Bhugra and Amit Malik.
Published by Cambridge University Press. © Cambridge University Press 2011.

1. **Case-focused assessments**: these are assessments that involve trainee performance in relation to an individual case (patient).
2. **Multi-source feedback**: this group of assessments is based on feedback from professional colleagues, and patients and their carers.
3. **Assessment of other professional activities**: this includes assessment of non-clinical skills related to professional and educational activities, such as journal-club presentations, written communications, chairing meetings, teaching and supervising other colleagues.

These three categories will next be considered in some detail. Commonly used assessment methods will be described alongside evidence from literature in relation to them.

Case-focused assessments

Case-focused assessments involve assessment of a trainee in relation to an individual patient. Depending on the type of assessment, trainees can be assessed and given feedback on the overall evaluation and management of a patient or on aspects of a patient's care. Some of the more universally utilized case-focused assessment methodologies are discussed here.

Long case assessment

Traditionally, the long case assessment has involved a trainee seeing an unstandardized patient in an unobserved setting to undertake a complete history and examination and then presenting the case to one or more examiners, followed by unstructured questioning by the examiners, in order to establish the trainee's skills. Generally, such cases take up to one hour of consultation, followed by thirty minutes of assessment.

Messages from literature

The long case assessment provides a truly authentic educational opportunity for an assessor to provide trainees with formative feedback on their ability to manage various aspects of individual cases. Pilot studies at the Royal College of Psychiatrists demonstrate that the ACE (assessment of clinical expertise) tool – which involves the trainee conducting a complete assessment of a real patient under the observation of a trained assessor – has reasonable feasibility and acceptability and indicates general ability (see Chapter 4).

Whilst the traditional long case assessment has many advantages, including authenticity, acceptability and educational value, its disadvantages, including non-generalizability, poor reliability and low validity, indicate that it is unsuitable for making high-stake decisions (Norcini, 2001). There are concerns with the reliability of the long case assessment because of its case specificity, the dependence on inter-rater reliability and the possibly limited range of competencies evaluated.

Many modifications of the long case assessment have been attempted, to enhance its psychometric properties and make it fit for the purpose of making high-stake decisions. Increasing the number of cases, using several assessors and having the trainee–patient interactions observed can help with some of these concerns (Ponnamperuma *et al.*, 2009). In addition, training the assessors to make accurate observations, using a particular tool or rating scale and providing action-orientated feedback will enhance the overall utility of the long case not only as a tool that can potentially be reliable enough to make high-stake decisions but also, more importantly, can be utilized for the overall development of the trainee (C. Fitch, A. Malik and P. Lelliott, personal communication, 2009). Developing clearly defined, authentic and validated anchor points for assessment tools and increasing the range of competencies assessed by the tools will also enhance the overall utility of long case assessment tools (Norcini, 2002).

Direct observation of procedural skills (DOPS)

Direct observation of procedural skills, that is, the observation of trainees whilst they undertake a practical procedure, enables the assessor to make judgements regarding the trainee's ability to carry out specific aspects of the procedure and the procedure as a whole (Wilkinson *et al.*, 2003). Generally, direct observation assesses technical procedures, such as intubation. Its role in psychiatry has been debated (Brown and Doshi, 2006). Direct observation can be used for physical treatment procedures, such as ECT, control and restraint, resuscitation and phys-ical examination. Some observers have argued that DOPS could be extended to specific tasks, such as assessing suicidal risks or a patient's suitability for cognitive behavioural therapy (CBT), but in these cases the additional advantage of using DOPS rather than mini-CEX or similar short focused assessments will need to be assessed and considered carefully.

Messages from literature

There is evidence of the reliability and validity of direct observation from its implementation for the assessment of the UK Foundation Programme trainees (Davies *et al.*, 2009), postgraduate medical trainees (Wilkinson *et al.*, 2008) and postgraduate psychiatric trainees (see Chapter 4).

Some important messages emanate from the application of DOPS or simi-lar instruments in other specialties and contexts. Observation checklists are less reliable than global rating scales (Martin *et al.*, 1997; Regehr *et al.*, 1998). How-ever, detailed checklists may serve a more useful formative purpose and can be utilized to give detailed and structured feedback. Additionally, procedural obser-vation tools are resource- and time-intensive, as the assessors need to be present during the procedure. Analysis of pilot data from the Royal College of Psychiatrists demonstrated the necessity to carry out a high number of observations to attain adequate reliability. This raises questions about its feasibility, although it is possible that this low reliability resulted from heterogeneity of assessor occupations (see Chapter 4). Evidence from the UK Foundation Assessment Programme (Davies *et al.*, 2009) and data obtained from medical trainees (Wilkinson *et al.*, 2008) also raise concerns regarding the time taken to undertake observations. However, the methodology does have reasonable user satisfaction. Therefore, the issue of time being made available to undertake DOPS must be addressed by assessment programme developers, especially if a high number of direct observations are recommended to support summative decisions. As stated before, data from the Royal College of Psychiatrists also emphasize the influence of observer occupation in the overall assessment outcomes (Chapter 4). This evaluation recommends using a spread of assessors, fixing the number of observations assessed by some occupational groups, such as consultant psychiatrists, as they provide a higher level of reliability. Finally, there have been concerns around observational errors committed by assessors; these concerns are not unique to DOPS and have also been raised with regards to other observational tools for decades (Holmboe *et al.*, 2003). However, with training, some of these observational errors can be reduced.

Mini-CEX (mini clinical evaluation exercise)

In addition to the mini-CEX, which was developed in the USA as a specific tool to counteract some of the challenges posed by the traditional long case assessment, this section also considers other assessment tools, such as the mini-ACE (mini assessed clinical encounter). In these methods, the trainee is directly observed by an assessor for approximately 20 minutes during a clinical encounter with a patient. During this time, the trainee's ability to undertake specific clinical tasks is assessed, whereas in the long case assessment every aspect of the trainee–patient encounter is assessed. Common examples in psychiatry include the assessment of components of the mental state, such as psychosis or suicidal risk.

A large body of evidence for the use of the mini-CEX comes from the American Board of Internal Medicine's application of this tool (American Board of Internal Medicine, 2002). More recently, the application of the tool in the Foundation Assessment Programme and some medical specialties in the UK has also helped us in our understanding of the mini-CEX (Davies *et al.*, 2009; Wilkinson *et al.*, 2008). A similar tool with fewer rating points and different domains, called the mini-ACE is also used in psychiatry in the UK (see Appendix 4.2).

Messages from literature

The mini-CEX has high internal consistency and reproducibility (Durning *et al.*, 2002; Kogan *et al.*, 2003). Previous studies have recommended the number of mini-CEXs that need to be carried out in certain specialties and contexts in order to facilitate high-stake decision-making. However, it is also possible to take a more pragmatic view and use the confidence intervals from a small number of mini-CEXs undertaken with the vast majority of trainees to decide whether further mini-CEXs are needed for borderline trainees, as has been shown in internal medicine (Norcini *et al.*, 1995; 2003). The other advantage of using the mini-CEX is that, since it does not take so long, it allows for sampling of a wider area of the curriculum than does the long case assessment.

The validity of the mini-CEX and the mini-ACE has also been demonstrated by correlation with other assessment methodologies, designed to assess similar constructs. Additionally, assessors are, to some extent, able to distinguish between different levels of standardized trainee performance (Holmboe *et al.*, 2003).

A single mini-CEX or mini-ACE ideally should take no more than 30 or 35 minutes and it is therefore felt to be a feasible assessment method. However, even with the short amount of time taken to carry out a mini-CEX, there are considerable overall time and resource implications both for clinical services and individuals (Davies *et al.*, 2009). Assessors tend to give high scores to their trainees, which indicates a further training need for the assessors (American Board of Internal Medicine, 2002). These high scores might also relate to the reluctance of assessors to mark down trainees whom they know well. Additionally, some trainees have difficulties in scheduling the mini-CEX in a busy workplace context (Morris *et al.*, 2006) and this is potentially a more generic problem with all workplace-based assessments. Finally, studies suggest that just because assessors observe trainees in this form of assessment, it does not actually imply that these observations are accurate, and observational errors do occur (Holmboe *et al.*, 2003).

To overcome these concerns, there are several suggestions in the literature. Firstly, using a wide spread of independent assessors and clinical cases allows both for triangulation of assessments and greater sampling of the curriculum (Wilkinson *et al.*, 2008). Secondly, there is a strong emphasis on assessor training, especially when it comes to observations and feedback (Holmboe *et al.*, 2003). Thirdly, with regards to the scheduling of these assessments and their ownership, it is suggested that these assessments should be compulsory and trainee-led with consequences for progression if these assessments are not carried out (Wilkinson *et al.*, 2008). Finally, some studies suggest that a standardized assessment tool with fewer and more clinically relevant domains, clear behavioural anchors, structured prompts and fewer levels on rating scales, may increase overall accuracy and the number of observations on the mini-CEX (Donato *et al.*, 2008).

Case-based discussion (CbD)

Case-based discussion (CbD) (or chart-stimulated recall, as it is commonly known in North America) involves the use of a written patient record to stimulate a discussion of the trainee's management, decision-making and note-keeping of a case and to provide specific feedback. Essentially, the trainee approaches the assessor with two or more clinical cases that the trainee has recently been involved in. The assessor then chooses one case and, using the trainee's recent entries in the patient's records as a focus point, leads a discussion regarding limited aspects of the case. This is then followed by assessor feedback. The entire process should typically take between 20 and 30 minutes.

Messages from literature

The CbD tool has adequate validity and reliability, as supported by reports from pilots of workplace-based assessments in psychiatric (see Chapter 4) and medical postgraduate training (Booth *et al.*, 2009) in the UK. This tool has high user satisfaction and popularity amongst trainees and assessors and can be feasibly implemented for formative purposes (Booth *et al.*, 2009). It also correlates with other assessment tools that purport to assess similar domains (Davies *et al.*, 2009). Evaluation of assessment programmes within different specialties in the UK highlights the fact that a varying number of CbDs are required, depending on the specialty and other contextual factors, to support high-stake decision-making (Booth *et al.*, 2009).

Notwithstanding the significant advantages of CbD and its high user acceptability, there are some concerns in implementing this tool. Firstly, there is evidence that the assessment can be influenced by the accuracy of trainees' recall and by their post-hoc rationalization of the case and management of it (Jennett and Affleck, 1998). It has been suggested that reducing the time between the trainee seeing a patient and the CbD might overcome some of this difficulty (Rubenstein and Talbot, 2003). There are also risks that the CbD can sometimes turn into a knowledge-based viva voce rather than the performance-based assessment that it is meant to be. Putting an emphasis on explanation and the decision-making process that the trainee utilizes in the management of the case and the manner in which this is reflected in the trainee's record-keeping might provide a truer picture of a trainee's performance and ability (Rubenstein and Talbot, 2003). As with other workplace-based assessment tools, assessor training significantly enhances the utility of the CbD. There is also evidence that a combination of the audit of patient charts (records) and CbD can be used to build a detailed picture of a clinician's performance (Nichols Applied Management, 2001).

Multi-source feedback (MSF)

Multi-source feedback can further be divided into feedback from professionals and feedback from users (patients) and their carers. The issues related to patient feedback on trainee performance are discussed in detail in Chapter 3, while this section focuses on feedback obtained from other professionals with whom the trainee works.

The term multi-source feedback describes a process rather than an individual assessment tool. It involves the assessment of a trainee's competence and behaviour from different perspectives, including their peers, supervisors, non-medical colleagues and patients. Its main benefits include assessments from several different viewpoints and the assessment of aspects of professional competence not assessed by other tools, such as humanistic and interpersonal skills. Various studies outline the number of reviewers required and this is influenced by the feedback and the clinical context. It is possible to achieve fairly high generalizability and reliability coefficients to support high-stake decision-making with many of the available MSF tools (Murphy *et al.*, 2009).

Multi-source feedback developers should arrive at an early consensus regarding the purpose of the feedback; this should be clearly communicated to all users, as a lack of clarity regarding purpose and practicalities can cause significant anxiety amongst users (Lockyer, 2003). There is now significant experience, described in the literature, of enhancing the content and construct validity of feedback tools (Hall *et al.*, 1999; Lelliott *et al.*, 2008). There is also evidence to support the importance of validating multi-source feedback within specialty-specific context (Davies *et al.*, 2008).

To ensure the successful implementation of multi-source feedback, logistic concerns of assessors, such as the excessive paperwork associated with providing ratings and giving feedback, must be addressed. This can be done in a variety of ways, including producing shorter instruments, centrally administering the feedback and using information technology (IT), not only to collect ratings but also to collate responses, so that supervisors can provide meaningful feedback.

Reviewer ratings depend on a complex range of factors, such as staff groups, seniority, interpersonal relations and the mood of the reviewer. Therefore, if feedback tools are to be used for making high-stake decisions, then these and other contextual cognitive and psychological factors must be taken into account to support reliable decision-making (Burford *et al.*, 2010). There is now considerable evidence regarding the variation in MSF ratings by individual staff or occupation groups. For instance, in one study, peers, administrators and managers were three or four times less likely to indicate concerns regarding junior doctors than consultants and senior nurses, who were more likely to express concerns, emphasizing the importance of clear guidance to trainees regarding the selection of assessors for feedback (Bullock *et al.*, 2009). There is, however, evidence that allowing trainees to choose their individual reviewers does not significantly influence the overall scores (Ramsey *et al.*, 1996).Therefore, whilst straight guidance must be issued regarding the occupational groups that provide ratings within a single feedback process, it might not be necessary to be didactic about the individuals who must complete this tool for a particular trainee. Such an approach also indicates the value of clear guidance and training for assessors.

Training in MSF tools is crucial not only for assessors but also for those providing feedback. However, there is evidence in the literature that acceptable inter-rater reliability can be achieved without specific training for some tools (Lelliott *et al.*, 2008). Different rater groups often focus on different aspects of professional competence. Therefore, poor inter-rater reliability, especially amongst different professional groups, may not always be a sign of poor psychometric properties of the tool. There have been many arguments to support the anonymity of assessors, but conventional wisdom now states that confidentiality is more important than anonymity, as it allows serious concerns to be investigated, and it also decreases the likelihood of fraudulent ratings by anonymous assessors.

The format and structure of feedback to the trainee is very important to ensure that multi-source feedback has a positive educational impact. Therefore, it is desirable that instead of trainees receiving collated ratings directly, these are sent to a supervisor who can discuss them with the trainee in a structured and meaningful manner and place the feedback in the context of the trainee's overall experience within the learning environment.

Whilst giving feedback, it is important to bear in mind the influence of emotions and reflection on feedback acceptance (Sargeant *et al.*, 2008). Furthermore, it is also important to recognise that trainees respond to feedback from different sources in different ways. For instance, medical trainees often focus on feedback from supervisors whilst minimizing the significance of feedback from non-medical colleagues (Higgins *et al.*, 2004). Additionally, participants' responses to feedback also differ, depending on the domains that assessors from different professional groups have assessed them on. As an example, in a study evaluating the performance ratings of practising interns by registered nurses, interns were more comfortable with nurses rating them on communication and humanistic skills than on their clinical care (Weinrich *et al.*, 1993). This raises two important issues. Firstly, assessors should be qualified to provide feedback on the domains that they are being asked to assess and, secondly, programme directors should make trainees aware of the importance of non-medical staff in clinical settings, especially in a truly multi-disciplinary profession, such as psychiatry. Interestingly, in a study looking at perception of MSF users, the trainees clearly expressed a preference for textual feedback, although the assessors preferred numerical scores. The users also felt that MSF was 'good in principle' but could not identify doctors in difficulty (Burford *et al.*, 2010).

In longitudinal studies, feedback scores have been shown to increase significantly, especially those scores that have been received from medical colleagues and co-workers (Violato *et al.*, 2008), although reasons for this may not be entirely clear. However, more work needs to be done with regards to the consequential validity of multi-source feedback, especially in determining the professional domains that can be best assessed by this format and, subsequently, in developing assessment tools that enjoy credibility within the profession (Sargeant *et al.*, 2007).

Assessment of other professional activities

In addition to the assessment methods described above, there are many other methods of assessment of different competencies contributing to the overall skill set of the trainee. In this final section some of these methods, which are used within and outside psychiatry, are outlined.

DONCS (direct observation of non-clinical skills)

This tool is an adaptation of the DOPS by the Royal College of Psychiatrists, and is designed to assess a trainee's non-clinical skills by observing them undertaking activities, such as chairing a meeting, teaching, supervising others, or engaging in non-clinical procedures. This tool is currently being piloted with senior psychiatric trainees across the UK (www.rcpsych.ac.uk).

JCP (journal-club presentations)

Journal clubs in psychiatric training are usually fora for trainees to meet regularly together with one or more consultants or specialists to discuss, in a structured manner, a particular paper published in a scientific journal. Usually one trainee critically evaluates a paper that has been previously circulated to the group and subsequently presents this evaluation to the entire group. This educational activity can be used to assess both the trainee's critical appraisal and presentation skills. There are many guidelines within the literature regarding the critical evaluation of papers (Greenhalgh, 1997) as well as the assessment of a trainee's presentation skills (Greenhalgh, 2006). However, literature regarding the assessment of journal-club presentations is sparse. The Royal College of Psychiatrists has evaluated these journal-club presentations in pilots of a journal-club presentation tool (see Appendix 4.7). Organizations in India, as well as in some other countries, have also used assessment of presentation skills.

Assessment of clinical letters

Written communication skills are an indispensable component of a trainee's overall competence, especially in the developed world. Evidence exists within other medical specialties that feasible and reliable methods can be developed to assess clinical letter writing as a proxy for the assessment of a trainee's written communication skills (Crossley et al., 2001). Detailed communication in psychiatry is best placed for such assessments.

Conclusion

This chapter has looked at some of the more commonly used traditional and contemporary assessment methods in psychiatry and medical education in general. Key research messages from the literature regarding some of these methods were discussed. A pragmatic classification of these tools has also been attempted in the hope that assessment programme developers will refer to all of this information when considering the use of several different assessment tools in an assessment programme. It is also anticipated that the acceptability for the assessment tools amongst their users will be enhanced if the evidence base around these assessment tools is more widely disseminated.

There are many other methods and tools not considered here, which have been developed locally. Some of these will be discussed in subsequent chapters, when assessment frameworks in different countries are considered. In the development of any such tools, basic principles should always be followed. Assessment tools should be components of an overall assessment programme supporting the curriculum; their purpose should be explicit and their utility should be evaluated within the context in which they will be applied.

REFERENCES

American Board of Internal Medicine (2002). *The Mini-CEX. A Quality Tool in Evaluation. Guidelines and Implementation Strategies from Program Directors.* Philadelphia: ABIM.

Booth, J., Johnson, G. and Wade, W. (2009). *Workplace-Based Assessment Pilot Report of Findings of a Pilot Study.* London: Royal College of Physicians.

Brown, N. and Doshi, M. (2006). Assessing professional and clinical competence: the way forward. *Advances in Psychiatric Treatment,* **12**, 81–91.

Bullock, A. D., Hassell, A., Markham, W. A., Wall, D. W. and Whitehouse, A. B. (2009). How ratings vary by staff group in multi-source feedback assessment of junior doctors. *Medical Education,* **43**, 516–520.

Burford, B., Illing, J., Kergon, C., Morrow, G. and Livingston, M. (2010). User perceptions of multi-source feedback tools for junior doctors. *Medical Education,* **44**, 165–176.

Crossley, J. G. M., Howe, A., Newble, D., Jolly, B. and Davies, H. A. (2001). Sheffield assessment instrument for letters (SAIL): performance assessment using outpatient letters. *Medical Education,* **35**, 1115–1124.

Davies, H., Archer, J., Bateman, A. *et al.* (2008). Specialty-specific multi-source feedback: assuring validity, informing training. *Medical Education,* **42**, 1014–1020.

Davies, H., Archer, J., Southgate, L. and Norcini, J. (2009). Initial evaluation of the first year of the Foundation Assessment Programme. *Medical Education,* **43**, 74–81.

Donato, A. A., Pangaro, L., Smith, C. *et al.* (2008). Evaluation of a novel assessment form for observing medical residents: a randomised, controlled trial. *Medical Education,* **42**, 1234–1242.

Durning, S. J., Cation, L. J., Markert, R. J. and Pangaaro, L. N. (2002). Assessing the reliability and validity of the mini-clinical evaluation exercise for internal medicine residency training. *Academic Medicine,* **77**(9), 900–904.

Greenhalgh, T. (1997). How to read a paper: assessing the methodological quality of published papers. *British Medical Journal,* **315**, 305–308.

Greenhalgh, T. (2006). *How to Read a Paper: The Basics of Evidence-Based Medicine.* Oxford: Blackwell.

Hall, W., Violato, C., Lewkonia, R. *et al.* (1999). Assessment of physician performance in Alberta: the Physician Achievement Review. *Canadian Medical Association Journal,* **161**(1), 52–57.

Higgins, R. S. D., Bridges, J., Burke, J. M. *et al.* (2004). Implementing the ACGME general competencies in a cardiothoracic surgery residency program using a 360-degree feedback. *Annals of Thoracic Surgery*, **77**, 12–17.

Holmboe, E. S., Huot, S., Chung, J., Norcini, J. and Hawkins, R. E. (2003). Construct validity of the mini clinical evaluation exercise (miniCEX). *Academic Medicine*, **78**(8), 826–830.

Jennett, P. and Affleck, L. (1998). Chart audit and chart stimulated recall as methods of needs assessment in continuing professional health education. *The Journal of Continuing Education in the Health Professions*, **18**, 163–171.

Kogan, J. R., Bellini, L. M. and Shea, J. A. (2003). Feasibility, reliability, and validity of the mini-clinical evaluation exercise (mCEX) in a medicine core clerkship. *Academic Medicine*, **78**(10), S33–S35.

Lelliott, P., Williams, R., Mears, A. *et al.* (2008). Questionnaires for 360-degree assessment of consultant psychiatrists: development and psychometric properties. *British Journal of Psychiatry*, **193**, 156–160.

Lockyer, J. (2003). Multisource feedback in the assessment of physician competencies. *The Journal of Continuing Education in the Health Professions*, **23**, 4–12.

Martin, J. A., Regehr, G., Reznick, R. *et al.* (1997). Objective structured assessment of technical skill (OSATS) for surgical residents. *British Journal of Surgery*, **84**, 273–278.

Morris, A., Hewitt, J. and Roberts, C. M. (2006). Practical experience of using directly observed procedures, mini clinical evaluation examinations, and peer observation in pre-registration house officer (FY1) trainees. *Postgraduate Medical Journal*, **82**, 285–288.

Murphy, D. J., Bruce, D. A., Mercer, S. W. and Eva, K. W. (2009). The reliability of workplace-based assessment in postgraduate medical education and training: a national evaluation in general practice in the United Kingdom. *Advances in Health Sciences Education*, **14**, 219–232

Nichols Applied Management (2001). *Alberta's Physician Achievement Review (PAR) Program: A Review of the First Three Years*. Report, Edmonton, Alberta: Nichols Applied Management.

Norcini, J. (2001).The validity of long cases. *Medical Education*, **35**, 720–721.

Norcini, J. J. (2002). The death of the long case? *British Medical Journal*, **324**, 408–409.

Norcini, J. J., Blank, L. L., Arnold, G. K. and Kimball, H. R. (1995). The mini-CEX (clinical evaluation exercise): a preliminary investigation. *Annals of Internal Medicine*, **123**(10), 795–799.

Norcini, J. J., Blank, L. L., Duffy, F. D. and Fortna, G. S. (2003). The mini-CEX: a method for assessing clinical skills. *Archives of Pediatrics and Adolescent Medicine*, **138**(6), 476–481.

Ponnamperuma, G. G., Karunathilake, I. M., McAleer, S. and Davis, M. H. (2009). The long case and its modifications: a literature review. *Medical Education*, **43**, 936–941.

Ramsey, P. G., Carline, J. D., Blank, L. L. and Wenrich, M. D. (1996). Feasibility of hospital-based use of peer ratings to evaluate the performances of practicing physicians. *Academic Medicine*, **71**(4), 364–370.

Regehr, G., MacRae, H., Reznick, R. K. and Szalay, D. (1998). Comparing the psychometric properties of checklists and global rating scales for assessing performance on an OSCE-format examination. *Academy of Medicine*, **73**, 993–997.

Rubenstein, W. and Talbot, Y. (2003). *Medical Teaching in Ambulatory Care*. New York: Springer.

Sargeant, J., Mann, K., Sinclair, D., Van Der Vleuten, C. P. M. and Metsemakers, J. (2007). Challenges in multisource feedback: intended and unintended outcomes. *Medical Education*, **41**, 583–591.

Sargeant, J., Mann, K., Sinclair, D., Van Der Vleuten, C. P. M. and Metsemakers, J. (2008). Understanding the influence of emotions and reflection upon multi-source feedback acceptance and use. *Advances in Health Sciences Education*, **13**, 275–288.

Violato, C., Lockyer, J. M. and Fidler, H. (2008). Changes in performance: a 5-year longitudinal study of participants in a multi-source feedback programme. *Medical Education*, **42**, 1007–1013.

Weinrich, M. D., Carline, I. D., Giles, L. M. and Ramsey, P. G. (1993). Ratings of the performances of practicing internists by hospital-based registered nurses. *Academic Medicine*, **68**, 680–687.

Wilkinson, J., Benjamin, A. and Wade, W. (2003). Assessing the performance of doctors in training. *BMJ*, **327**(7416), s91–s92.

Wilkinson, J. R., Crossley, J. G. M., Wragg, A. *et al.* (2008). Implementing workplace-based assessment across the medical specialties in the United Kingdom. *Medical Education*, **42**, 364–373.

3

Assessing the patient perspective

Jim Crossley

Editors' introduction

Whilst there is universal agreement that patients and their carers must be engaged in all aspects of healthcare development and delivery, this does not always happen in real life. This involvement of users and carers is even poorer when it comes to postgraduate psychiatric education, including the assessment of psychiatric trainees. In this precise discourse, Crossley presents a compelling evidence-based case, not only highlighting the significance of seeking patient feedback, but also strongly suggesting that feedback can be accessed feasibly, reliably and validly. He also discusses special considerations for seeking patient feedback within psychiatry and outlines some areas for relevant future research.

Introduction

Earlier chapters have argued that workplace-based assessment adds value to traditional assessment methods in two ways:

1. It allows for the assessment of complexity – the integrated application of knowledge, skills and attitudes to authentic clinical challenges. (This is the competency agenda, which has helped us to move away from artificial silos of knowledge, skill and attitude (McClelland, 1973)).
2. It allows for the assessment of real day-to-day performance – the highest point of Miller's helpful pyramid (Miller, 1990). This matters because a clinician's competence (the best he or she is capable of) is a poor predictor of real day-to-day performance (Rethans *et al.*, 2002). If you want to know what actually happens day to day, you have to assess in the workplace.

Of course, for every advantage there are always disadvantages. The uncontrolled nature of the workplace means that every clinician is assessed on different

Workplace-Based Assessments in Psychiatric Training, ed. Dinesh Bhugra and Amit Malik.
Published by Cambridge University Press. © Cambridge University Press 2011.

challenges by different assessors – and we know that case differences and judge differences have a substantial influence on performance scores (Crossley *et al.*, 2002). Also, the communities of assessors in the workplace are not highly trained specialists. They should know about what they're being asked to judge, but they don't usually all have a full understanding of the purpose and background of the assessment, and they may have very different standards. The assessment isn't their main job, and they may even bring their own agenda to the assessment process in such a way that it is undermined.

When we ask patients to assess their clinicians in the workplace, we play to all the strengths of WPBA, and we play to all of its weaknesses. The remaining sections of this chapter will fill out the implications of this statement. I know of no peer-reviewed publications evaluating a patient rating instrument in a psychiatric setting. Indeed, the most recent review of patient survey and feedback instruments found none that was validated for use in a psychiatric setting (Evans *et al.*, 2007). However, there is some unpublished research evaluating the application of a generic patient rating instrument across several specialties, including psychiatry. The findings of this study are cited with the investigators' permission. The lack of evidence means that this chapter will be a brief commentary rather than a lengthy review.

Throughout the chapter, the traditional term patient is used for simplicity – acknowledging that many readers will be more comfortable or familiar with the terms 'service user' or 'client'.

Why the patient's view matters

Only patients can judge certain aspects of performance

There are very many reasons why we should be interested in the patient's perspective on his or her care. They fall into three main themes:
1. The patient is the clinician's customer and society is the clinician's employer.
2. The patient's engagement in the relationship is fundamental to therapeutic success.
3. The patient has a unique and important perspective on the clinician's performance.

The third reason is the most important from a workplace-based assessment perspective: this type of assessment is all about gaining an insight into clinicians' authentic performance and patients are uniquely placed to provide that insight. Patients see things that no colleague sees; this may include excellent and dangerous practice. Also, just as colleagues are best able to judge whether a clinician displays the necessary clinical and technical performance, so patients are the experts on certain aspects of relational performance, such as building trust or listening properly. Patients also consistently report that these are the elements of their care about which they feel most strongly (Elwyn *et al.*, 2007).

In the context of psychiatry, there can be a very particular power imbalance between doctor and patient. From the extreme situation in which a psychotic patient cannot be depended upon to act in his or her own best interests, to the more subtle situations in which patients with dementia or personality disorders may need to be given boundaries for their safety and for the safety of others, the family, the doctor and other professionals may assume power over patients. With power comes the potential for abuse. In this context, it is vital that the patient's view is heard – albeit through careful filters – since the patient may be the only one aware of the abuse. To fail to listen to a vulnerable patient with a mental health problem is unforgivable. It is like failing to listen to a child who is suffering abuse.

Clinicians care what their patients think about them

Another interesting finding outside psychiatry is that doctors are very highly sensitive to what their patients think of them. In appraisal discussions, doctors are prone to accept the validity of their patient ratings even though they frequently challenge the validity of their colleagues' ratings.

In summary, patient ratings are important because patients are the only authentic experts on certain elements of a clinician's performance, because patients see things that no-one else sees, and because doctors are responsive to patients' feedback.

The hazards of patient ratings in psychiatry

Small case-loads may not allow for sufficiently wide sampling

I have already acknowledged that judges frequently have different standards (varying stringency) and different perspectives on what constitutes good performance (subjectivity). This is as true of patients as judges as it is of colleagues or other 'professional' observers. Moreover, attempts to turn judgements into objective responses fail to solve the problem. Either the assessment is distorted so that only a formulaic performance is judged as 'good' – this is called 'futility' – or the final assessment performs less precisely or discriminatingly (less reliably) than the 'subjective' one. Rather than trying to turn subjective judgements into objective responses, we must acknowledge subjectivity and ensure that we sample enough judges' views adequately to reflect the views of the whole spectrum of judges. Generalizability analysis can quantify the contribution that judges' subjectivity makes to the spread of ratings and allows us to calculate how many responses are required to reflect adequately the views of all judges. When we apply this kind of analysis to patient ratings in other settings, we typically find that 20 or more responses are required. In a psychiatric context, clinicians frequently have small active case-loads. This makes it challenging to recruit sufficient respondents to achieve reliable results.

Put simply, the contribution that an idiosyncratic patient makes to the overall rating is disproportionate if only a small number of patients provide ratings.

Patients may struggle to identify the contribution of each clinician

Most studies of patient ratings highlight the fact that patients struggle to identify who they are rating and to what extent the clinician in question has contributed to their overall care (Rodriguez *et al.*, 2009). Psychiatrists frequently work in multi-disciplinary teams including therapists, psychiatric nurses, social workers, the primary care team, and others. This makes it especially difficult to 'extract' the contribution of the psychiatrist to perceived success or failure. Indeed, in some settings, those aspects of care about which patients feel most strongly – such as listening and support – may be devolved to other members of the mental health team very deliberately.

Mental illness may affect the reliability of responses

Most clinicians feel nervous about asking patients to comment on the care that they provide. Those insecurities are even greater with psychiatric patients, who may be unreliable respondents because of the nature of their condition. Patients with dementia frequently struggle to identify individuals close to them and are even more likely to struggle in identifying a particular clinician. Disorders of affect strongly influence responses acquired from patients in a wide range of questionnaire-based surveys; there is no reason why a nihilistic perspective should not have a similar effect on performance ratings. Psychotic illness seems likely to influence patients' responses in unpredictable ways. Persecutory delusions, for example, provide a poor basis for a balanced judgement about care. Patients with personality disorders carry both intrinsic idiosyncrasies in their views of other people (including their psychiatrists) and they are prone to reactive tensions in their relationships: they are more likely to generate confrontational or dependent interactions and they are able to take advantage of fewer life-chances. Both these factors will affect the way in which they perceive the performance of the health professionals who work with them.

Atypical clinician–patient relationships may distort responses

Over and above unreliable responses, some psychiatric patients may be strategically deviant responders. Forensic psychiatrists do not have a normal relationship with their patients; indeed the relationship may be adversarial. Some patients may use ratings in the same way that they use complaints – to undermine the credibility of a psychiatrist who has provided an unfavourable assessment.

Empirical findings from published data outside psychiatry

Patient ratings are feasible in a range of settings

Feasibility evaluations have concluded that, despite challenges, patients can be encouraged to provide ratings of their doctor's performance for education and assessment purposes in both primary and secondary care settings. In general, these work better if a third party is specifically employed to administer the question-naire or instrument and if responses are collected 'on the spot' rather than posted back later (Crossley *et al.*, 2008). There is no empirical comparison between the reliability and validity of assessments in which doctors select their own patient respondents, and assessments in which a third party makes this selection – but, in most settings, it would seem more appropriate for a third party to select respon-dents, to avoid selection bias.

Patients can provide reproducible and discriminating ratings

Given the fact that patients are being asked to make subjective judgements, it is reassuring to know that, outside psychiatry, an assessment that samples sufficient patients' views is reliable. For example, using one validated patient rating instru-ment, comparing doctors on the basis of one respondent's rating each, the score spread is much more strongly influenced by the particular patient respondent than by the doctor (reliability coefficient 0.18). Comparing doctors on the basis of 20 patients' responses each, the score spread is more than 80% dependent on the doctors (reliability coefficient 0.81) (Crossley *et al.*, 2005).

The pattern of responses across items suggests that they are meaningful

Also, the internal structure (intercorrelations) of responses suggests that respon-dents are able to use discrete items on a questionnaire-based instrument in a meaningful way. Administering an instrument designed to measure the five con-structs 'interpersonal skills', 'patient-centredness', 'child-centredness', 'information gathering' and 'information giving' to the parents of children in paediatric con-sultations, their responses to items within each construct correlate much more strongly than their responses across constructs. These correlation patterns are sufficiently strong that the factor structure suggests that parents are rating four separate latent variables. Those variables are almost perfectly matched to the five constructs (Crossley *et al.*, 2005).

Patients and colleagues independently agree about clinicians' relational performance

Finally, whilst the overall ratings of colleagues and the overall ratings of patients do not correlate across doctors (because they are assessing different aspects of performance), colleagues ratings of a doctor's relational performance display a significant correlation with the ratings provided completely blindly and indepen-dently by their patients (Crossley *et al.*, 2008). This provides extremely compelling evidence of the validity of both patients' and colleagues' ratings.

Some groups are too idiosyncratic to be reliable

However, there are some groups of respondents who do not provide reliable ratings – in the sense that they are not consistent with each other. In the study quoted above, both children and their parents were asked to rate the doctor's performance. Whilst the aggregated ratings of 20 parents provided a precise and discriminating measure of one doctor's performance compared with another, children – rating the same consultations – were so inconsistent between them that even the aggregated scores of 100 children did not produce a reliable measure of one doctor compared with another (Crossley *et al.*, 2005). Inconsistency between them does not, of course, invalidate the child's view of the interaction. Most doctors would want to know what any patient perceived from the interaction, however idiosyncratic. But it does mean that aggregated individual responses are not able to generalize to reflect a doctor's performance with any patient.

Empirical findings from unpublished studies within psychiatry

In 2007, the Academy of Medical Royal Colleges (AoMRC) commissioned from the Royal Colleges of Physicians (RCP) an evaluation of two generic WPBA instruments across all specialties in the UK. This evaluation was in response to the recommendation of the Chief Medical Officer that re-licensure might be underpinned by an assessment using a generic multi-source feedback (MSF) system applicable to the vast majority of doctors in the UK (Department of Health, 2007). One instrument was designed for professional colleagues to rate a doctor's performance. The other instrument was designed for patients to rate a doctor's performance. The patient rating instrument is presented in Appendix 3.1.

The findings of that evaluation are still being prepared for publication. However, some aspects of the evaluation are highly relevant to this chapter and these are discussed below with the kind permission of the authors.

Feasibility

Participants were recruited from 14 specialties by writing to the Royal Colleges and asking them to invite members and fellows to participate. On this basis, 73 psychiatrists volunteered to participate. This was the third largest cohort of any specialty. Of those 73 psychiatrists, 48 (66%) were able to obtain ratings from more than 20 patients within a limited timescale. This is similar to the other specialties. On the basis of recruitment and response rates, it would appear that patient ratings are at least as easy to gather in psychiatry as in any other specialty.

Reliability

Patient respondents in psychiatry showed a noticeably different score pattern from the other 13 specialties. Psychiatrists received the lowest mean ratings. Also, a far

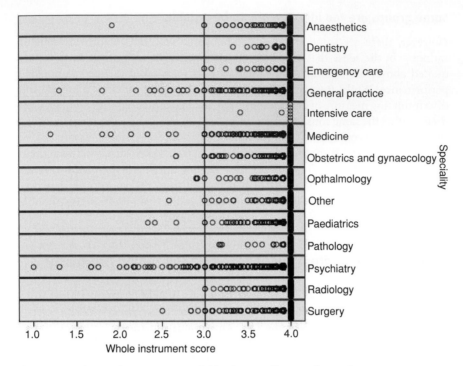

Figure 3.1 Patient rating across 14 specialties (scatter diagram of scores)

greater proportion of patients responded 'not really' or 'definitely not' to positive descriptions of their psychiatrist (below 3 on the scatter diagram – Figure 3.1) than patients in any other specialty. Interestingly however, there was considerable consistency between patients rating the same psychiatrist, so that a psychiatrist viewed critically by one patient tended to be viewed critically by most patients and vice versa. Consequently, of the four specialties with sufficient participants to estimate reliability (general practice, medicine, paediatrics and psychiatry), patient ratings for psychiatry proved to be the most reliable.

Validity

Certain items on the generic AoMRC instrument produced idiosyncratic results in psychiatry. Item 6 (which asks, 'Are you involved as much as you want to be in the decisions about your care and treatment?') and item 10 (which asks, 'By the end of the consultation did you feel better able to understand and/or manage your condition and your care?') were rated significantly lower by psychiatric patients than by patients in other specialties. Items 9.1 and 9.2 (which ask about examination) were less frequently completed than in other specialties. Given the nature of psychiatry, these response patterns could be judged to provide positive evidence for the validity of responses; they are patterns that might be predicted if patients are using the questions meaningfully. However, they also raise doubts about whether a 'generic' patient ratings instrument can offer the best means for patients to provide and doctors to receive feedback concerning psychiatric interactions. As with many other specialist jobs (Davies *et al.*, 2008), it is almost certainly more helpful to use a bespoke instrument for psychiatry that highlights the most important elements of performance in interactions.

Implications for implementation

1. The vulnerability of psychiatric patients and the feasibility and reliability of psychiatric patient ratings in the AoMRC evaluation form suggest that patient ratings should and probably can be used to assess psychiatrists in the workplace.
2. As with all disciplines, the purpose of patient ratings must be clear to all concerned, and should drive the way in which the scores are handled.
3. There is evidence that psychiatric patients, as a group, can provide valid and reliable responses. However, the problems associated with psychiatric patients and the clinical interaction mean that each response requires filtering – just as the responses from child respondents require filtering. Consequently, it is probably not appropriate to use raw mean ratings to compare one psychiatrist with another. Also, the high proportion of 'unsatisfactory' responses means that one or two such responses should not automatically trigger concern about a psychiatrist's interactions without further corroborating evidence or some confidential consideration of the type of patient(s) providing the response(s). This is materially different from other specialties, where two unsatisfactory responses from patients provide a good predictor of a doctor being in difficulty.
4. It should be recognized that some psychiatrists may not be able to participate in patient rating assessments because of the nature of their case-loads.
5. Like other specialty areas, bespoke patient ratings instruments will probably provide more meaningful performance information than generic instruments, such as the one presented in Figure 3.1. There are a good number of bespoke instruments in circulation but none appears to have been evaluated empirically.

Implications for research

1. A systematically derived description of the key performance elements in a psychiatric consultation should inform the content of any patient rating instrument. Appropriate methods include an empirical approach, such as interaction process analysis, or a consensus approach, such as a Delphi exercise. Any consensus approach should include patients as equal partners with clinicians.
2. Whilst patients' ratings have been shown to be reliable in reproducibly discriminating between clinicians in the quoted evaluation, this finding needs further

investigation. Firstly, a larger-scale evaluation is required with an instrument specifically designed for psychiatric interactions. Secondly, the psychiatric sub-specialty should be included in the explanatory model. It is possible that reliable distinctions between psychiatrists are actually a function of their sub-specialty and not of the relational ability of the psychiatrist. Put simply, all the stringently rated psychiatrists may have been working in forensic psychiatry and their stringent ratings may reflect the nature of their respondent group.

3. Just as parents provide the most reliable ratings of doctors consulting with their children, so other carers and family members may provide valid and reliable proxy responses for certain psychiatric patients – such as those with dementia or psychotic disorders. This requires evaluation.

APPENDIX 3.1 PATIENT RATING INSTRUMENT

What did you think of this doctor?	Yes, Definitely	Yes, to some extent	Not Really	Definitely Not	Does not apply
1. Was the doctor polite and considerate?	☐	☐	☐	☐	☐
2. Did the doctor listen to what you had to say?	☐	☐	☐	☐	☐
3. Did the doctor give you enough opportunity to ask questions?	☐	☐	☐	☐	☐
4. Did the doctor answer all your questions?	☐	☐	☐	☐	☐
5. Did the doctor explain things in a way you could understand?	☐	☐	☐	☐	☐
6. Are you involved as much as you want to be in the decisions about your care and treatment?	☐	☐	☐	☐	☐
7. Did you have confidence in the doctor?	☐	☐	☐	☐	☐
8. Did the doctor respect your views?	☐	☐	☐	☐	☐
9. If the doctor examined you, did he or she:					
a. Ask your permission?	☐	☐	☐	☐	☐
b. Respect your privacy and dignity?	☐	☐	☐	☐	☐
10. By the end of the consultation did you feel better able to understand and/or manage your condition and your care?	☐	☐	☐	☐	☐

11. Overall, how satisfied were you with the doctor you saw?

Very Satisfied ☐   Fairly Satisfied ☐   Not Really Satisfied ☐   Not at all Satisfied ☐

Please make any additional comments about the doctor in the space below
Please remember that this is just about the doctor you have seen today

<u>About You – The Patient</u>

Gender		Age	
Male	☐	Under 16	☐
Female	☐	16 - 30	☐
Who is Filling out this form?		31 - 45	☐
You – the patient	☐	46 - 60	☐
Family member or carer	☐	61 - 75	☐
Facilitator	☐	76 +	☐
Interpreter	☐	Prefer not to say	☐
Is English your first language? Yes ☐ No ☐			

REFERENCES

Crossley, J., Humphris, G. and Jolly, B. (2002). Assessing health professionals. *Medical Education*, 36(9), 800–804.

Crossley, J., Eiser, C. and Davies, H. (2005). Children and their parents assessing the doctor–patient interaction: a rating system for doctors' communication skills. *Medical Education*, 39(8), 820–828.

Crossley, J., McDonnell, J., Cooper, C. *et al.* (2008). Can a district hospital assess its doctors for re-licensure? *Medical Education*, 42(4), 359–363.

Davies, H., Archer, J., Bateman, A. *et al.* (2008). Specialty specific multi-source feedback–assuring validity, informing training. *Medical Education*, 42(10), 1014–1020.

Department of Health (2007). *The White Paper Trust, Assurance and Safety: The Regulation of Health Professionals*. London: The Stationery Office.

Elwyn, G., Buetow, S., Hibbard, J. and Wensing, M. (2007). Respecting the subjective: quality measurement from the patient's perspective. *BMJ*, 335, 1021–1022.

Evans, R. G., Edwards, A., Evans, S., Elwyn, B. and Elwyn, G. (2007). Assessing the practising physician using patient surveys: a systematic review of instruments and feedback methods. *Family Practice*, 24, 117–127.

McClelland, D. C. (1973). Testing for competence rather than for 'intelligence'. *American Psychologist*, 28, 1–14.

Miller, G. E. (1990). The assessment of clinical skills/competence/performance. *Academic Medicine*, S63–S67.

Rethans, J.-J., Norcini, J. J., Baron-Maldonado, M. *et al.* (2002). The relationship between competence and performance: implications for assessing practice performance. *Medical Education*, 36(10), 901–909.

Rodriguez, H. P., von Glahn, T., Chang, H., Rogers, W. H. and Safran, D. G. (2009). Measuring patients' experiences with individual specialist physicians and their practices. *American Journal of Medical Quality*, 24, 35–44.

4

Experience of workplace-based assessment in the UK

Andrew Brittlebank

Editors' introduction

Developments in the evidence base for assessing postgraduate training and the establishment of a new regulatory body for postgraduate medical education provided impetus for change in the manner in which postgraduate trainees are assessed in the United Kingdom. In this chapter, Brittlebank not only discusses the socio-political context in which these changes were introduced and implemented in a top-down manner, but also provides quantitative and qualitative measures associated with specific workplace-based assessment tools and their implementation in the UK. He also outlines the importance of such initiatives as user training and development of electronic systems to reduce the bureaucratic burden of assessments. Finally, he emphasizes the importance of utilizing the assessments to contribute to a culture of continual development. He believes that this will happen if, in addition to focusing on the psychometric properties of performance-based assessments, efforts are made to enhance their acceptability amongst their end-users.

Introduction

In this chapter, I will sketch the history of the introduction and development of workplace-based assessment (WPBA) in psychiatry training in the UK. It is an interesting story, containing many elements: WPBA was initiated at the insistence of the statutory regulator; it was taken up enthusiastically by a group of 'early adopters' within the Royal College of Psychiatrists and it has raised a number of concerns. Among the issues raised are fears that WPBA will herald the end of formal examinations and thus will lead to a 'dumbing down' of professional

Workplace-Based Assessments in Psychiatric Training, ed. Dinesh Bhugra and Amit Malik. Published by Cambridge University Press. © Cambridge University Press 2011.

standards (Oyebode, 2009; Sikdar, 2010), concerns that WPBAs will unhelpfully encroach on processes of educational supervision (Julyan, 2009), worries about the administrative burden of delivering WPBAs (Babu *et al.*, 2009) and, finally, reports that trainees hold 'negative attitudes' towards WPBA (Menon *et al.*, 2009).

Along the way, I will outline some of the findings from studies that have evaluated the use of workplace-based assessments in UK psychiatry. The first of the studies was a small field trial in a single healthcare provider, the second study was a large-scale pilot study that involved a number of sites around the UK and there was also a small qualitative study that aimed to explore what was happening in the hearts and minds of psychiatric trainees involved in the change from an assessment system based on examinations and supervisor reports to one that included workplace-based assessment.

The author is grateful to Dr Julian Archer of the Peninsula Medical School for the statistical analysis of the pilot data.

Background

The introduction of workplace-based assessments in the UK took place in the context of a major structural and cultural reform of postgraduate medical education that began in the early years of the new millennium. Prior to this, the pattern of postgraduate medical education (PGME) in the UK had not changed since the inception of the UK's National Health Service (NHS) in 1948 and was regulated by the medical royal colleges and largely based upon an apprenticeship model.

The medical royal colleges are bodies that have their origins in the eighteenth century. According to Downie and Charlton (1992), the colleges' original purpose was to protect the monopolistic interests of their members, which they did through controlling entry to specialist practice by setting examinations for membership and fellowship. The Royal College of Psychiatrists is one of the more recently formed medical royal colleges, being constituted in its present form in 1971. Prior to that most UK psychiatrists passed the examination for membership of the Royal College of Physicians or held a Diploma in Psychological Medicine granted following examination by a university. After its foundation, the Royal College of Psychiatrists followed the pattern of the other medical royal colleges by setting its own membership examination, which the trainee doctor had to pass before being allowed to proceed to higher training as a specialist registrar. Higher training continued for a further three to four years, after which the specialist registrar was entitled to apply for a senior career-grade post as an NHS consultant psychiatrist, or senior specialist.

Typically, trainee specialist doctors in the UK would spend the early part of their specialist training in a series of short-term posts. Training in these posts was poorly coordinated and they were not a part of recognized training programmes with clear training goals. Doctors in such posts were poorly supervised, poorly assessed and appraised, and did not have access to career advice. As a group, they contributed disproportionately to service and received little in the way of training benefit. The state of affairs was such that, collectively, the grade was widely described as 'the workhorses of the NHS' and the 'lost tribe' (Dillner, 1993).

The first official criticism of this method of organizing postgraduate medical education came in 2002 in a discussion paper entitled 'Unfinished business' written by Sir Liam Donaldson, the Chief Medical Officer for England.

Modernising Medical Careers (Department of Health, 2003) was the programme that was initiated following the consultation. It proposed a new structure for postgraduate training progression along with major changes in the culture of PGME. It was fully implemented in 2007.

The major structural change was the organization of all junior doctor posts into programmes of training. For the individual doctor, this begins with the two-year Foundation Training Programme, which doctors are to undertake following graduation and prior to embarking on a six-year specialty training programme, leading to eligibility to apply for senior specialist posts. The cultural change was to signal a move away from the apprenticeship approach of the trainee 'serving time', and being subject to infrequent 'high-stake' assessments in the form of examinations and job interviews. In the new approach, trainees are to gain carefully supervised experiences, in which they demonstrate prescribed competencies before progressing to the next stage of development.

At the same time as the above changes took place, a new body, the Postgraduate Medical Education and Training Board (PMETB) was constituted as the statutory regulator of postgraduate medical education in the UK and it assumed many of the responsibilities that were held by the medical royal colleges. The PMETB asked the colleges to develop curricula and assessment systems and stipulated a number of standards that they must fulfil (PMETB, 2009). Implicit in this, the PMETB indicated that assessment systems must be embedded in training and that trainee specialists must participate in frequent 'low-stake' assessments in the workplace.

The changes in postgraduate medical education led to the development and evaluation of a number of workplace-based assessment programmes in the UK, focused on different medical specialties and different stages of training. For example, the Royal College of Physicians evaluated the use of four different WPBA tools for trainees in internal medicine (Wilkinson *et al.*, 2008). Davies *et al.* (2009) reported an evaluation of a programme of workplace-based assessments for doctors in the first two years of postgraduate practice. The broad conclusions from these studies were that WPBA programmes can be feasibly introduced to postgraduate medical education in the UK and that the tools have some validity and reliability in the settings in which they were studied.

The initial field trial

Although the results of the studies were encouraging, none of the studies involved psychiatric trainees. There was a need to test the WPBA methods in psychiatry training.

We therefore conducted a small-scale field trial of the use of some WPBA tools in psychiatry (Brittlebank, 2007). This study was conducted in a single mental health provider organization that employed 35 junior trainees in psychiatry. The tools that were tested were the mini-clinical evaluation exercise (mini-CEX), the case-based discussion (CbD) and the direct observation of procedural skills (DOPS). These tools were selected because there was already some familiarity with them; they had been used for two years in pilot studies of workplace-based assessment in the Foundation Training Programme. The study found that psychiatry trainers and trainees were able to use the tools and to complete them within existing time constraints, and they found them to be acceptable methods of assessment. Trainees reported that it was not always convenient for them to be assessed and they complained abut the burden of paperwork that the WPBAs placed on them.

The field trial also revealed that the tools did not cover all the identified needs of psychiatric training. In particular there was an unmet need for a tool that would assess a full clinical encounter; the WPBA equivalent of the 'long case' examination. It was recommended that some of the existing tools be modified to better meet the needs of psychiatry and new instruments were developed.

The UK national pilot study

In August 2006, the Royal College of Psychiatrists led a national pilot study to evaluate the new tools that had been developed for psychiatric training, as well as those that had been adapted from the Foundation Programme. The Royal College pilot study also gave the opportunity of evaluating the assessment tools' performance in assessing trainees' progress against the version of the curriculum that was then available.

The tools that were the subjects of this evaluation were: directly observed procedural skills (DOPS), the mini assessed clinical encounter (mini-ACE) (adapted from the mini-CEX), the assessment of clinical expertise (ACE) (the WPBA equivalent of the 'long case'), case-based discussion (CbD), multi-source feedback (MSF), patient satisfaction questionnaire (PSQ), clinical presentation (CP) and journal-club presentation (JCP).

Description of tools

The evidence base for most of the tools described below has been discussed in greater details elsewhere in this volume. However, it might be prudent, in addition to describing the assessment tools utilized in the pilot, also to briefly outline their background. All these assessment tools (with the exception of the patient satisfaction questionnaire, which requires further development) are attached in the appendices at the end of this chapter.

The direct observation of procedural skills (DOPS) was developed by the Royal College of Physicians in the UK to be a tool to assess a trainee's performance of practical procedures, such as venepuncture or intubation (Wilkinson *et al.*, 2003). Early psychometric data on the DOPS in internal medicine suggests that the reliability and validity of this instrument compares favourably with the data for the mini-CEX (Wilkinson *et al.*, 2008). The main use for this in psychiatry is in assessment of the performance of ECT. The assessor watches the trainee performing the procedure, including communication with the patient and other members of the healthcare team. The assessment therefore provides an opportunity to give feedback on the trainee's humanistic skills as well as technical skill (Appendix 4.1).

The mini assessed clinical encounter (mini-ACE) is based on the mini clinical evaluation exercise (mini-CEX) (Norcini *et al.*, 1995). Previous studies of the mini-CEX in internal medicine indicate that it has good reliability (Kogan *et al.*, 2003) and validity (Holmboe *et al.*, 2003). The mini-ACE involves an assessor watching the trainee perform part of the clinical encounter, such as history taking. It takes about 20 minutes to conduct (Appendix 4.2).

The assessment of clinical expertise (ACE) is the equivalent of the clinical evaluation exercise (CEX). It may be thought of as a WPBA equivalent of the 'long case' examination. The CEX has been reported to have low reliability (Norcini, 2002) but the approach has a great deal of face validity to psychiatrists (Brittlebank, 2007). The ACE involves an assessor observing an entire clinical encounter, which should ideally be a new patient assessment. This instrument may assess a full range of patient assessment and treatment skills (Appendix 4.3).

The CbD is similar to the 'chart-stimulated recall', in which the assessor conducts an interview of a trainee based on what the trainee has written in a patient's clinical record. The interview allows an exploration of all aspects of the trainee's clinical reasoning (Appendix 4.4). There are few studies of the psychometric properties of this tool (Davies *et al.*, 2009; Fitch *et al.*, 2008).

The mini-PAT is a multi-source feedback tool developed for medical trainees to gather assessments from co-workers (Archer *et al.*, 2008). It is based on the Sheffield Peer Review Assessment Tool (SPRAT), which has been shown to have good feasibility and construct validity data (Archer *et al.*, 2005). The mini-PAT has been shown to have good reliability, validity and feasibility when studied in the UK Foundation Programme (Davies *et al.*, 2009) and in UK training programmes for internal medicine (Wilkinson *et al.*, 2008).The trainee asks approximately 12 colleagues to anonymously rate his or her performance, at the same time, the trainee completes a self-rating. The aggregated ratings of co-workers are compiled and compared with the trainee's self-ratings (Appendix 4.5).

The patient satisfaction questionnaire is a novel patient feedback tool, to gather patient assessments of psychiatric trainees. It was designed to allow patients to rate a trainee's humanistic skills and behaviours such as politeness, listening skills, or answering questions. The trainee asks 12 patients to complete the forms anonymously and send them back to a central point for collation of aggregated scores. Although a number of tools have been developed to enable patients to give feedback on the performance of their doctors, none has been developed to be used for psychiatrists in training and only two, the Physician Achievement Review (PAR) and the Sheffield Patient Assessment Tool (SHEFFPAT), have been subjected to reasonably rigorous reliability and feasibility studies (Chisolm and Askham, 2006). These studies indicated that around 25 patient responses were needed to provide reliable data on a doctor's performance (Crossley *et al.*, 2005; Violato *et al.*, 2003).

The case presentation (CP) is another novel tool developed by the UK Royal College of Psychiatrists. It was introduced to assess a trainee's performance in presenting cases at 'grand rounds' or other clinical educational meetings on which they would not have been previously assessed in a structured way (Searle, 2007). The assessor (usually the chairperson of the meeting) is asked to rate the trainee's performance in four areas: the clinical assessment of the patient, the trainee's interpretation of the clinical material, the use of investigations, and the trainee's presentation and delivery (Appendix 4.6).

The JCP (journal-club presentation) is also a novel tool developed by the UK Royal College of Psychiatrists. It was introduced alongside the CP (Searle, 2007) and is intended to assess a trainee's performance in presenting at journal clubs. The assessor (usually the chairperson of the meeting) assesses the trainee's performance on a number of domains, including introducing the topic, analysis and critique of evidence, presentation and delivery, and answering questions. (Appendix 4.7)

These assessment tools were administered singly and in various combinations to trainee psychiatrists across 16 pilot sites, taking in approximately 600 psychiatric trainees. The pilot sites consisted of a range of psychiatric training schemes that varied in size from small rotations of 10 specialty trainees (STs) to large deanery-wide schemes of up to 100 STs. The training schemes are drawn from England, Scotland and Wales and represent both urban and rural localities as well as teaching hospital and non-teaching hospital and community-based clinical services.

Training in WPBA was delivered on the pilot sites, so that each site was offered a three-hour training package that covered the elements of assessor training that Holmboe *et al.* (2004) identified as being necessary to improve the quality of assessments, that is performance dimension training, observational ratings and frame-of-reference training.

Quantitative aspects

The assessment forms that were used in the pilot sites were printed on multi-part carbonless paper, which produced two copies of each assessment. The trainee retained the bottom copy of the assessment form and the top copy was read by document recognition software. The software then produced summary reports for each assessment tool that was used in the pilot.

The study evaluated the reliability of the individual tools using generalizability theory, which is a means of systematically identifying and quantifying errors of measurement in educational tests. In a well-designed and controlled study, it is possible to include in the analysis the effects of various factors, such as the assessors, clinical setting or occasions, to determine how much each contributes to measurement error. Analyses of the intercorrelations between assessment tools were undertaken to explore the relationships in performance across the assessment programme, in order to support or refute evidence for validity and to inform the future development of the assessment programme. The acceptability and feasibility of the tools were evaluated by asking assessors and trainees to rate their satisfaction with the episode of assessment on a Likert-type scale graded from 1 to 6 and to record the time taken to complete the assessment.

The generalizability data showed that several of the instruments were capable of providing reliable standards of assessment at feasible numbers of assessments. Indeed, some of them achieved the levels of reliability regarded as necessary for 'high-stake' assessments. The case-based discussion produced a highly reliable assessment after an average of 100 minutes of assessment with four assessors; the assessed clinical encounter after 185 minutes with five assessors and the mini-ACE after 192 minutes with eight assessors. The mini-PAT and patient satisfaction questionnaire produced appropriate levels of reliability and precision for multi-source feedback tools from six and five assessors, respectively. The findings for the case-based discussion, assessed clinical encounter and mini-ACE were comparable to the findings using similar instruments in studies of other groups of medical trainees in the UK (Archer *et al.*, 2005; Davies *et al.*, 2009; Wilkinson *et al.*, 2008).

The DOPS, case presentation and journal-club presentation were found to have such low reliability scores that they could not produce reliable and precise assessment scores within a feasible number of assessments. The reliability of the DOPS in this study was much lower than found in other studies (Davies *et al.*, 2009; Wilkinson *et al.*, 2008). This may have been due to the heterogeneity of the assessors, where nurses and other junior doctors performed many of the assessments.

The results of this study presented good evidence for the validity of the assessment instruments. All the instruments that included a measure of user satisfaction were rated highly by trainees and assessors. All the instruments apart from the patient satisfaction questionnaire included a global rating of trainee performance. The global ratings were highly correlated with the aggregate of the other scores, indicating a high degree of criterion validity. Further reassurance for the validity of the instruments is provided by the high correlations between the instruments.

The patient satisfaction questionnaire was the exception to the above observations about validity. In this study, trainees' scores on the PSQ did not correlate with any of the other instruments. This may be taken as evidence of lack of validity for the PSQ; alternatively, it may be claimed that patients have a unique perspective on psychiatrist performance, which needs to be taken into account. Clearly, more work is needed in the area of patient feedback in assessing psychiatrists in training.

Because the study included data from a large number of trainees who had been assessed using several instruments, it allowed the opportunity to explore the relationships between the assessment tools.

Trainees' scores on the case and journal-club presentations were found to be highly correlated, raising the possibility that the tools assess the same construct, namely presentation skills. It may therefore be reasonable to combine the results of these assessments into a single score. If this is done, a highly reliable and precise assessment is produced from an average of 150 minutes' assessment time with six assessors.

The assessed clinical encounter and mini-ACE were also found to be highly correlated. Furthermore, there was a strong similarity between the instruments in the diagnostic groups assessed and the profile of assessors who completed them, and it also emerged that the time taken to complete the two assessments was not significantly different. These findings support the argument to drop one of the tools. If this is done, this could lead to a saving of approximately one and a half hours of assessment time.

The results of the study also raised implications for the nomination and training of assessors. The majority of the case-focused assessments (ACE, mini-ACE and CbD) were performed by senior specialists (consultant psychiatrists). Such assessors were found to produce more reliable and precise assessments than other assessors. Nursing staff and other junior doctors, particularly those closest in seniority to the doctor being assessed, tended to provide much more lenient assessments than their senior medical counterparts. This supports the argument for constraining the ability of trainees to nominate large numbers of non-consultants as assessors. Alternatively, if other assessors, particularly non-medical colleagues are to continue to assess, they will need targeted training in appropriate assessment standards.

These findings from the initial pilot study provided reassurance that much of the psychiatry assessment system is valid and can feasibly produce reliable and precise assessments. Further work is needed to produce a form of assessment that reliably and validly incorporates the patient's viewpoint. Decisions are needed concerning combining the assessments of presentation skills and using one tool to assess observed clinical encounters.

Qualitative aspects

As well as evaluating the strict psychometric qualities of the WPBA tools, we also wanted to explore subtle aspects of the impact of the introduction of the tools on psychiatric trainees. To that end, we conducted a small qualitative study at one of the pilot sites that had been using WPBA tools for more than a year.

The study recruited interviewees from among the psychiatry trainees employed in one mental health provider and asked them to talk about their experience of the new form of assessment. While it would have been ideal to conduct a naturalistic study of the everyday talk of participants, this was not possible for both practical and ethical reasons. Six trainees were recruited into the study, consisting of two from each of the first three years of psychiatric training and there were equal numbers of male and female trainees.

The protocol for this study received ethical approval from the appropriate institutional research ethics committee.

Trainees who participated in this study were given the choice to be interviewed anonymously, over the telephone, by a senior psychiatric trainee or face-to-face by a chartered clinical psychologist.

The semi-structured interview was designed following the guidance provided by Smith (1995). The purpose of the interview was to explore participants' experience of WPBA and to encourage them to talk about their views of the various types of assessment.

The interviewers made an audio recording of each interview, from which a transcription was prepared. Participants were given copies of their interview transcripts, to check their accuracy and to give an opportunity to withdraw material from the study, should they so wish. The transcripts were then subject to a thematic analysis.

Many of the trainees mentioned that the introduction of WPBA had transferred the responsibility for organizing aspects of their work experience and their assessments from their senior colleagues to the trainees. That is, it becomes the trainee's responsibility to organize their work strategically so that they could have the balance of experiences that best increased their prospects of getting the right assessments. For example, a male trainee recounted how in his work so far he had not been expected to perform electroconvulsive therapy (ECT), but after seeing that he needed to demonstrate competency in this technique in order to progress to the next stage of training, he arranged to swap duties with a colleague, so that he could get the required competency 'signed off'.

However, the organization of work to meet the needs of assessment may operate in the opposite direction, to make trainees reluctant to undertake some clinical tasks that no longer meet their strategic needs. Such tasks, including phlebotomy, which is seen as menial, and performing assessments at night, which are seen as intrusive on rest time, can be left for other staff to perform, once the trainee has achieved competence in them.

Trainees spoke of time pressures to maintain the assessment schedule. In her interview, one female trainee commented several times about the need for trainees 'to be organized' in order to complete the required number of assessments within the guidelines and to 'keep up to date' with their assessments.

Trainees also talked of the burden they felt in having to take the initiative in organizing episodes of assessment, even when senior colleagues were not willing or available to make the assessment. Trainees need to be vigilant for opportunities to be assessed. As another doctor said:

So what I do is grab the opportunity: one example is that I've had only one or two home visits and one knows that it's very rare for trainees to make frequent home visits, so I grabbed an opportunity, and I was with the senior social worker, and when we went back to the base I just asked if he could fill the [assessment] form in.

While it was apparent that the trainee psychiatrists interviewed found the WPBA process anxiety provoking and an inconvenience, they were able to identify some benevolent aspects:

It is a hassle, but it's a good hassle, because if you don't do it, you won't know where you are...

There was evidence that trainees saw the assessments as a positive opportunity to develop their professional skills and knowledge. Commenting on the effects of being assessed as performing at the expected level for the current stage of training, one trainee commented:

You want to do more so that you meet the level above your expectation, so that's what you strive for.

A number of trainees commented that the new assessment tools were helpful because they indicated when they had achieved competence and thereby allowed the trainee to take pride in the demonstration of a particular skill.

Trainees spoke of the tools being helpful 'to identify and correct weaknesses' and to 'refine and polish' particular skills. For one doctor they also provided reassurance:

... they [the assessments] are marked highly in most domains; all it says to you is keep doing what you're doing. Maybe that's the message that you might need to hear: 'Please keep doing what you're doing.'

Some trainees, especially those who had several years of experience, contrasted the new workplace-based methods positively with former methods of assessment. The major contrasting system was that of the supervisor's six-monthly report, which was largely based on the supervisor's global impression of the trainee. Trainees described the new system as 'fairer', 'objective' and 'focused'. One trainee described another positive effect of the new system:

I don't feel that I'm being marked all the time, which is something I have felt on previous jobs, not psychiatric jobs, more in medical school. In placements in medical school where you didn't have very structured assessments, you were constantly trying to impress, which is irritating to everyone else and it's stressful for you.

Trainees also valued the opportunity to be given feedback and a few noted how assessments supported their self-reflection and contributed to learning planning:

It's for the trainees, good feedback for them... you're given feedback and you know where you stand.

On the first supervision session you discuss your learning objectives, you discuss what your strengths and weaknesses are... and after the third month and sixth month you review things and see whether you were able to improve, you get feedback from your consultant and the forms... it has been helpful to reflect on how much you feel you've improved.

But this was not a universal view as one trainee said:

Yes, it [being assessed in the workplace] helps in terms of getting someone to look at your competency... It's very objective, but does it actually make a difference? That's open to question.

An unexpected finding emerged from one or two trainees, who commented on the effect of being assessed by non-medical members of the multi-disciplinary team. It would appear that they saw their openness to being assessed by members of other professions as a source of validation.

One doctor talked of the legitimization he experienced as a result of being positively assessed by non-psychiatric members of his work team:

It allows me to be assertive when I disagree with them [members of other professional groups] because I know that they've signed a bit of paper that says I'm competent. . . . I think the fact that you're open to scrutiny: I know where I stand, I know that they think I'm competent or better, or whatever.

The legitimization process extended to the trainee's relationship with senior colleagues and a questioning of the senior's legitimacy. For example, a trainee commented that there were situations in which she felt that the assessment process enabled her to question the competence of her trainer:

The feedback he [my trainer] gave – I thought wasn't appropriate for my level of training . . . I wondered if it was appropriate for him to be doing an assessment of me. At that point I had some doubts in my mind that maybe he should have had more training before he could give feedback to me.

The live workplace-based assessment system

For six months prior to the launch of the assessment system, the College was involved in an intensive process of delivering training in WPBA methods around the country. A total of 40 training events were held in venues in all the English regions, in Wales, Scotland and Northern Ireland. A total of 1500 psychiatrists attended these events. In addition, training materials were developed for trainers to give to colleagues. As a result of this strategy, national surveys of medical trainers have shown that psychiatry trainers were better prepared for the introduction of workplace-based assessment than their colleagues in other medical disciplines (for example, see PMETB, 2009).

The College's new assessment system was approved by PMETB and went 'live' in August 2007, with the full implementation of *Modernising Medical Careers*. The assessment system was designed to sample all levels of medical competence, as described by Miller (1990). The system therefore included WPBA tools to assess the doctor's performance. There would be a national examination that consisted of three written papers, testing the psychiatrist's knowledge base and a clinical examination made up of 16 objective structured clinical examination (OSCE) stations, designed to test the psychiatrist's competence.

The WBPA tools consisted of those that had been used in the national pilot study, apart from the patient feedback tool (patient satisfaction questionnaire). The patient satisfaction questionnaire was not included because its scores failed to correlate with other aspects of the assessment system and it was decided that it needed further development before it could be recommended.

The College commissioned an online assessment provider to make the administration and storage of WPBA tools easier. For a number of reasons, including the need to have the assessment tools more clearly branded as College material and to have greater control over the use of the assessment data, the College brought the administration of the online WPBA tools 'in-house' after a year.

In the time since the system went live there have been three studies that have looked at various consequences of the workplace-based assessment system.

The first study was an exploration of the effects that workplace-based assessment had on the trainees' relationships with their trainers, or educational supervisors (Julyan, 2009). This is an important question because this relationship is a key part of a trainee's experience. It was felt that there could be a conflict of interest for the educational supervisors in providing objective assessments for trainees with whom they also had mentoring relationships. Despite finding that a significant amount of supervision time was being used to conduct WPBA, the study found no evidence that doing so detracted from the supervision relationship.

The second study was a questionnaire-based survey of the attitudes of psychiatry trainees in one geographical area to the introduction of workplace-based assessment (Menon *et al.*, 2009). This study revealed that while most trainees surveyed believed that WPBA had been introduced for good educational reasons and valued the feedback they received from senior colleagues, there was a great deal of mistrust of the tools and the technology supporting them. The authors' concerns about the technology were only partly answered by the College's decision to bring the system in-house. The greatest source of resentment for the trainees surveyed was the fact that they were being asked to pay for the assessment system.

The final study was also located in a single area of the UK, but it looked at the reactions of both trainers and trainees to the introduction of WPBA (Babu *et al.*, 2009). This study was much more positive. A very high proportion of the trainers surveyed (88%) had been trained in the use of WPBA and they expressed very positive attitudes towards the process. The trainees were much less positive, with fewer than 40% regarding WPBA as a useful way to help them prepare for clinical practice. Many saw assessment as a hindrance, and, as with the second study, they had experienced difficulty using the previous online provider's system.

Discussion

The introduction of workplace-based assessment into UK psychiatry is one aspect of an ongoing change in the culture of postgraduate training. We are changing from a situation in which assessment is something conducted in a distant examination centre, to one in which assessment is embedded in everyday work. The nature of the assessment is also changing, from infrequent high-stake pass-or-fail tests, to formative assessments that are intended to be part of a continuing process of development. The evidence suggests that the change that is required to the assessment culture is only happening slowly.

We can be assured from the results of pilot studies that WPBA can produce assessments that are valid and reliable. Indeed, in some respects, the reliability of some of the WPBA tools exceeds that of some aspects of traditional examinations.

As always, the most important issues are not about the objective findings, in this case the psychometric data of WPBA. Instead, the issues are about perceptions; that is, the hearts and minds of the people involved.

As would be expected, the main findings from the small qualitative study revealed that trainees have had a range of different experiences and hold a number of views about WPBA. The views are considered and nuanced. Some of these findings accorded with later studies (Babu *et al.*, 2009; Menon *et al.*, 2009), for example, comments about the need for WPBA systems to be user-friendly and not to overburden trainees. The trainees who were interviewed, however, seemed to have a greater appreciation of the place of WPBA in good educational practice, such as providing opportunities for receiving feedback and guiding further learning. This finding may be due to the different methodologies of data collection, in that the interviews allowed a deeper exploration of viewpoints than that permitted by a questionnaire. Alternatively, it may be due to differences of experience of WPBA. Trainees in the pilot-study sites had the same access to WPBA training as their senior colleagues did and this may have gone some way to allaying the fears that trainees had.

What lessons does this offer for other countries that are considering introducing a system of WPBA into their psychiatry training?

Firstly, development of the tools and gathering data about their psychometric properties should go hand in hand with training the end-user. This is necessary to ensure that the tools selected have validity for the psychiatrists involved and it is a necessary part of winning hearts and minds.

Secondly, the system for recording and storing the results of the assessment must be designed around the user. It is vital that the systems must not only be secure, but that they must also be based on readily accessible technologies and be user-friendly.

Thirdly, and most importantly, the purposes of WPBA must be clearly stated and presented to trainees as well as trainers.

Finally, assessment systems can only be useful if they contribute to a culture of continual improvement, both of individual doctors and of healthcare systems. It was interesting that WPBA led one of our interviewees to express doubt about the competence of her senior clinicians. If the process of WPBA can permit the expression of such doubts as part of an ongoing conversation between colleagues of different levels of seniority, then the medical culture will truly have changed. As has been said by one group of medical education experts, 'these techniques (of WPBA) reinforce an educational culture in which feedback for learning is the norm' (PMETB, 2009, p. 6).

APPENDIX 4.1 ASSESSMENT SHEET FOR DOPS

Trainee's GMC Number ☐☐☐☐☐☐☐ **DOPS** Date of Assessment ☐☐☐☐**20**☐☐
Surname: Forename:

Direct Observation of Procedural Skills (DOPS) ST All levels

RC
PSYCH
ROYAL COLLEGE OF
PSYCHIATRISTS

Setting: **Gen. Hosp**☐ **OPD**☐ **In-patient** ☐ **Crisis/ Emergency**☐ **CMHT** ☐

ST level of trainee:☐

	Below standard for end of ST level			Meets standard for ST level completion	Above expected ST level standard		
	1	2	3	4	5	6	u/c
1. Understanding of indications etc.	☐	☐	☐	☐	☐	☐	☐
2. Obtains informed consent	☐	☐	☐	☐	☐	☐	☐
3. Appropriate preparation	☐	☐	☐	☐	☐	☐	☐
4. Appropriate analgesia/ sedation	☐	☐	☐	☐	☐	☐	☐
5. Technical ability	☐	☐	☐	☐	☐	☐	☐
6. Aseptic technique	☐	☐	☐	☐	☐	☐	☐
7. Seeks help where appropriate	☐	☐	☐	☐	☐	☐	☐
8. Post-procedure management	☐	☐	☐	☐	☐	☐	☐
9. Communication skills	☐	☐	☐	☐	☐	☐	☐
10. Consideration/professionalism	☐	☐	☐	☐	☐	☐	☐
11. Overall ability	☐	☐	☐	☐	☐	☐	☐

12. Based on this assessment, how would you rate the Trainee's performance at this stage of training?

	Below expectations			satisfactory	better than expected		u/c
	☐	☐	☐	☐	☐	☐	☐

Anything especially good?	Suggestions for development

Agreed action:

Assessor's position: Consultant ☐ SASG ☐ Psychologist ☐ Nurse (Band 6 or above) ☐
Other ☐ (Profession: Seniority:)
Assessor's signature......

Please print Assessor's name......

Assessor's Registration number ☐☐☐☐☐☐☐☐   Date:

APPENDIX 4.2 ASSESSMENT SHEET FOR MINI-ACE

Mini-Assessed Clinical Encounter (Mini-ACE)CT1 Level

RC PSYCH
ROYAL COLLEGE OF
PSYCHIATRISTS

Trainee

Name:
Test Trainee

GMC Number:
Not Specified

Training Level:
CT1

Assessment Details

Date of assessment:

Focus of assessment (tick all that apply)

- [ ] Assessment of a psychiatric emergency (acute psychosis)
- [ ] Assessment of change in functioning
- [ ] Assessment of a common psychiatric condition
- [ ] Assessment of a complex psychiatric condition
- [ ] Assessment of response to treatment
- [ ] Assessment of a severe and enduring mental illness
- [ ] Assessment of a psychiatric emergency (suicidal feelings and acts)
- [ ] Management of a psychiatric emergency (acute psychosis)
- [ ] Management of a common psychiatric condition
- [ ] Management of a complex psychiatric condition
- [ ] Management of a severe and enduring mental illness
- [ ] Management of a psychiatric emergency (suicidal feelings and acts)
- [ ] Obtaining informed consent
- [ ] If the focus of the assessment is not listed above then please describe it here

| Clinical Setting | [ ] General Hospital | [ ] OPD | [ ] In-patient | [ ] Crisis/Emergency |
| | [ ] CMHT | [ ] Other (Please Specify) | | |

| Prev Contact | [ ] 0 | [ ] 1-4 | [ ] 5-9 | [ ] >9 |

| Complexity | [ ] Low | [ ] Average | [ ] High |

Diag 1: F

Diag 2: F

Mini-Assessed Clinical Encounter (Mini-ACE)CT1 Level

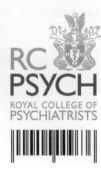

RC
PSYCH
ROYAL COLLEGE OF
PSYCHIATRISTS

Trainee

Name:
Test Trainee

GMC Number:
Not Specified

Training Level:
CT1

Assessment gradings

Please use the following rating scale:

1-3	Below standard for end of CT1
4	Meets standard for CT1 completion
5-6	Above CT1 standard
U/C	Unable to Comment

	1	2	3	4	5	6	U/C
1. History taking	☐	☐	☐	☐	☐	☐	☐
2. Mental State examination	☐	☐	☐	☐	☐	☐	☐
3. Communication skills	☐	☐	☐	☐	☐	☐	☐
4. Clinical judgement	☐	☐	☐	☐	☐	☐	☐
5. Professionalism	☐	☐	☐	☐	☐	☐	☐
6. Organisation/Efficiency	☐	☐	☐	☐	☐	☐	☐
7. Overall clinical care	☐	☐	☐	☐	☐	☐	☐
8. Based on this assessment, how would you rate the Trainee's performance at this stage of training?	☐	☐	☐	☐	☐	☐	☐

Assessment Comments

Anything especially good

Suggestions for development

Agreed action

APPENDIX 4.3 ASSESSMENT SHEET FOR ACE

Assessment of Clinical Expertise (ACE)CT1 Level

RC
PSYCH
ROYAL COLLEGE OF
PSYCHIATRISTS

Trainee

Name:
Test Trainee

GMC Number:
Not Specified

Training Level:
CT1

Assessment Details

Date of assessment:

Focus of assessment (tick all that apply)

- [ ] Assessment of a psychiatric emergency (acute psychosis)
- [ ] Assessment of change in functioning
- [ ] Assessment of a common psychiatric condition
- [ ] Assessment of a complex psychiatric condition
- [ ] Assessment of response to treatment
- [ ] Assessment of a severe and enduring mental illness
- [ ] Assessment of a psychiatric emergency (suicidal feelings and acts)
- [ ] Management of a psychiatric emergency (acute psychosis)
- [ ] Management of a common psychiatric condition
- [ ] Management of a complex psychiatric condition
- [ ] Management of a severe and enduring mental illness
- [ ] Management of a psychiatric emergency (suicidal feelings and acts)
- [ ] Obtaining informed consent
- [ ] If the focus of the assessment is not listed above then please describe it here

Clinical Setting	☐ General Hospital	☐ OPD	☐ In-patient	☐ Crisis/Emergency
	☐ CMHT	☐ Other (Please Specify)		
Prev Contact	☐ 0	☐ 1-4	☐ 5-9	☐ >9
Complexity	☐ Low	☐ Average	☐ High	

Diag 1: F

Diag 2: F

Assessment of Clinical Expertise (ACE)CT1 Level

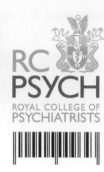

RC
PSYCH
ROYAL COLLEGE OF
PSYCHIATRISTS

Trainee

Name:
Test Trainee

GMC Number:
Not Specified

Training Level:
CT1

Assessment gradings

Please use the following rating scale:

	1-3	Below standard for end of CT1
	4	Meets standard for CT1 completion
	5-6	Above CT1 standard
	U/C	Unable to comment

	1	2	3	4	5	6	U/C
1. History taking	☐	☐	☐	☐	☐	☐	☐
2. Mental State examination	☐	☐	☐	☐	☐	☐	☐
3. Communication skills	☐	☐	☐	☐	☐	☐	☐
4. Clinical judgement	☐	☐	☐	☐	☐	☐	☐
5. Professionalism	☐	☐	☐	☐	☐	☐	☐
6. Organisation/Efficiency	☐	☐	☐	☐	☐	☐	☐
7. Overall clinical care	☐	☐	☐	☐	☐	☐	☐
8. Based on this assessment, how would you rate the Trainee's performance at this stage of training?	☐	☐	☐	☐	☐	☐	☐

Assessment Comments

Anything especially good

Suggestions for development

Agreed action

APPENDIX 4.4 ASSESSMENT SHEET FOR CBD

Case-based Discussion (CbD)CT1 Level

RC
PSYCH
ROYAL COLLEGE OF
PSYCHIATRISTS

Trainee

Name:
Test Trainee

GMC Number:
Not Specified

Training Level:
CT1

Assessment Details

Date of assessment:

Focus of assessment (tick all that apply)

- [ ] Assessment of a psychiatric emergency (acute psychosis)
- [ ] Assessment of change in functioning
- [ ] Assessment of a common psychiatric condition
- [ ] Assessment of a complex psychiatric condition
- [ ] Assessment of response to treatment
- [ ] Assessment of a severe and enduring mental illness
- [ ] Assessment of a psychiatric emergency (suicidal feelings and acts)
- [ ] Management of a psychiatric emergency (acute psychosis)
- [ ] Management of a common psychiatric condition
- [ ] Management of a complex psychiatric condition
- [ ] Management of a severe and enduring mental illness
- [ ] Management of a psychiatric emergency (suicidal feelings and acts)
- [ ] Obtaining informed consent
- [ ] If the focus of the assessment is not listed above then please describe it here

Clinical Setting	☐ CMHT	☐ Crisis/Emergency	☐ General Hospital	☐ In-patient
	☐ OPD	☐ Other (Please Specify)		
Prev Contact	☐ 0	☐ 1-4	☐ 5-9	☐ >9
Complexity	☐ High	☐ Average	☐ Low	

Diag 1: F

Diag 2: F

Case-based Discussion (CbD)CT1 Level

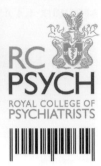

RC
PSYCH
ROYAL COLLEGE OF
PSYCHIATRISTS

Trainee

Name:
Test Trainee

GMC Number:
Not Specified

Training Level:
CT1

Assessment gradings

Please use the following rating scale:

1-3	Below standard for end of CT1
4	Meets standard for CT1 completion
5-6	Above CT1 standard
U/C	Unable to Comment

	1	2	3	4	5	6	U/C
1. Clinical record keeping	☐	☐	☐	☐	☐	☐	☐
2. Clinical assessment/diagnosis	☐	☐	☐	☐	☐	☐	☐
3. Risk assessment/management	☐	☐	☐	☐	☐	☐	☐
4. Medical treatment	☐	☐	☐	☐	☐	☐	☐
5. Investigation and referral	☐	☐	☐	☐	☐	☐	☐
6. Follow-up/care planning	☐	☐	☐	☐	☐	☐	☐
7. Professionalism	☐	☐	☐	☐	☐	☐	☐
8. Clinical decision making	☐	☐	☐	☐	☐	☐	☐
9. Overall clinical care	☐	☐	☐	☐	☐	☐	☐
10. Based on this assessment, how would you rate the Trainee's performance at this stage of training?	☐	☐	☐	☐	☐	☐	☐

Assessment Comments

Anything especially good

Suggestions for development

Agreed action

APPENDIX 4.5 ASSESSMENT SHEET FOR MINI-PAT

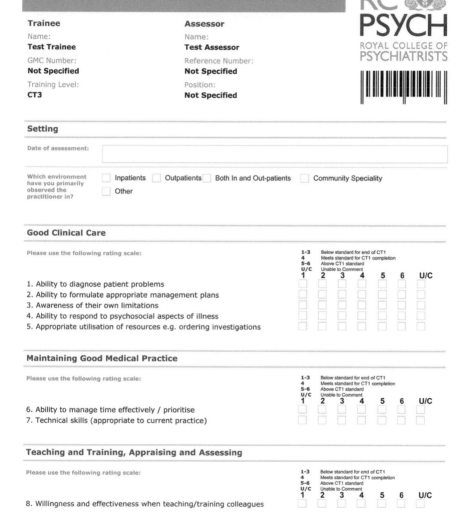

Mini-Peer Assessment Tool (Mini-PAT)CT1 Level

RC
PSYCH
ROYAL COLLEGE OF
PSYCHIATRISTS

Trainee	Assessor
Name:	Name:
Test Trainee	**Test Assessor**
GMC Number:	Reference Number:
Not Specified	**Not Specified**
Training Level:	Position:
CT3	**Not Specified**

Setting

Date of assessment:

Which environment have you primarily observed the practitioner in?
☐ Inpatients ☐ Outpatients ☐ Both In and Out-patients ☐ Community Speciality
☐ Other

Good Clinical Care

Please use the following rating scale:

1–3 Below standard for end of CT1
4 Meets standard for CT1 completion
5–6 Above CT1 standard
U/C Unable to Comment

	1	2	3	4	5	6	U/C
1. Ability to diagnose patient problems	☐	☐	☐	☐	☐	☐	☐
2. Ability to formulate appropriate management plans	☐	☐	☐	☐	☐	☐	☐
3. Awareness of their own limitations	☐	☐	☐	☐	☐	☐	☐
4. Ability to respond to psychosocial aspects of illness	☐	☐	☐	☐	☐	☐	☐
5. Appropriate utilisation of resources e.g. ordering investigations	☐	☐	☐	☐	☐	☐	☐

Maintaining Good Medical Practice

Please use the following rating scale:

1–3 Below standard for end of CT1
4 Meets standard for CT1 completion
5–6 Above CT1 standard
U/C Unable to Comment

	1	2	3	4	5	6	U/C
6. Ability to manage time effectively / prioritise	☐	☐	☐	☐	☐	☐	☐
7. Technical skills (appropriate to current practice)	☐	☐	☐	☐	☐	☐	☐

Teaching and Training, Appraising and Assessing

Please use the following rating scale:

1–3 Below standard for end of CT1
4 Meets standard for CT1 completion
5–6 Above CT1 standard
U/C Unable to Comment

	1	2	3	4	5	6	U/C
8. Willingness and effectiveness when teaching/training colleagues	☐	☐	☐	☐	☐	☐	☐

Mini-Peer Assessment Tool (Mini-PAT)CT1 Level

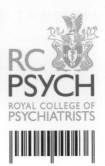

RC PSYCH
ROYAL COLLEGE OF
PSYCHIATRISTS

Trainee	Assessor
Name:	Name:
Test Trainee	**Test Assessor**
GMC Number:	Reference Number:
Not Specified	**Not Specified**
Training Level:	Position:
CT3	**Not Specified**

Relationship with Patients

Please use the following rating scale:

1-3   Below standard for end of CT1
4   Meets standard for CT1 completion
5-6   Above CT1 standard
U/C   Unable to Comment

	1	2	3	4	5	6	U/C
9. Communication with patients	☐	☐	☐	☐	☐	☐	☐
10. Communication with carers and/or family	☐	☐	☐	☐	☐	☐	☐
11. Respect for patients' dignity and their right to privacy & confidentiality	☐	☐	☐	☐	☐	☐	☐

Working with colleagues

Please use the following rating scale:

1-3   Below standard for end of CT1
4   Meets standard for CT1 completion
5-6   Above CT1 standard
U/C   Unable to Comment

	1	2	3	4	5	6	U/C
12. Verbal communication with colleagues	☐	☐	☐	☐	☐	☐	☐
13. Written communication with colleagues	☐	☐	☐	☐	☐	☐	☐
14. Ability to recognise and value the contribution of others	☐	☐	☐	☐	☐	☐	☐
15. Accessibility/reliability	☐	☐	☐	☐	☐	☐	☐

Global Ratings and Concerns

Please use the following rating scale:

1-3   Below standard for end of CT1
4   Meets standard for CT1 completion
5-6   Above CT1 standard
U/C   Unable to Comment

	1	2	3	4	5	6	U/C
16. Overall, how do you rate this trainee compared to others at the same grade?	☐	☐	☐	☐	☐	☐	☐
17. How would you rate the Trainee's performance at this stage of training?	☐	☐	☐	☐	☐	☐	☐

Health and probity

Do you have any concerns about this practitioner's health in relation to their fitness to practice   ☐ Yes   ☐ No

Mini-Peer Assessment Tool (Mini-PAT)CT1 Level

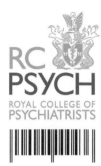

RC
PSYCH
ROYAL COLLEGE OF
PSYCHIATRISTS

Trainee

Name:
Test Trainee

GMC Number:
Not Specified

Training Level:
CT3

Assessor

Name:
Test Assessor

Reference Number:
Not Specified

Position:
Not Specified

Health and probity continued...

If yes please state your concerns:

Do you have any concerns about this practitioner's probity?   ☐ Yes   ☐ No

If yes please state your concerns:

Do you have any additional comments   ☐ No   ☐ Yes

Any additional comments

APPENDIX 4.6 ASSESSMENT SHEET FOR CASE PRESENTATION

Trainee's GMC Number ☐☐☐☐☐☐☐ **CP** Date of Assessment ☐☐☐☐20☐☐
Surname: Forename:

Case Presentation - eg Grand Round (CP) ST All levels

RC PSYCH
ROYAL COLLEGE OF PSYCHIATRISTS

ST level of trainee: ☐ *Diag*: F ☐☐ F ☐☐ F ☐☐ *Complexity*: **low** ☐ **mod** ☐ **high** ☐

	Below standard for end of ST level			Meets standard for ST level completion	Above expected ST level standard		
	1	2	3	4	5	6	u/c
1. Assessment and clinical examination	☐	☐	☐	☐	☐	☐	☐
2. Interpretation of clinical evidence	☐	☐	☐	☐	☐	☐	☐
3. Use of investigations	☐	☐	☐	☐	☐	☐	☐
4. Presentation and delivery	☐	☐	☐	☐	☐	☐	☐
5. Global rating	☐	☐	☐	☐	☐	☐	☐

6. Based on this assessment, how would you rate the Trainee's performance at this stage of training?

Below expectations			satisfactory	better than expected		u/c
☐	☐	☐	☐	☐	☐	☐

Comments:

Assessor's position: Consultant ☐ SASG ☐ Psychologist ☐ Nurse (Band 8 or above) ☐
Other ☐ (Profession: Seniority:)
Assessor's signature......

Please print Assessor's name......

Assessor's Registration number ☐☐☐☐☐☐☐☐   Date:

APPENDIX 4.7 ASSESSMENT SHEET FOR JCP

Trainee's GMC Number ☐☐☐☐☐☐☐ **JCP**   Date of Assessment ☐☐☐☐**20**☐☐

Surname: Forename:

Journal Club Presentation (JCP) **ST All levels**	RC PSYCH ROYAL COLLEGE OF PSYCHIATRISTS

ST level of trainee: ☐ *Diag*: F ☐☐ F ☐☐ F ☐☐   *Complexity*: **low** ☐ **mod** ☐ **high** ☐

	Below standard for end of ST level			Meets standard for ST level completion	Above expected ST level standard		
	1	2	3	4	5	6	u/c
1. Introducing the topic	☐	☐	☐	☐	☐	☐	☐
2. Setting material in context	☐	☐	☐	☐	☐	☐	☐
3. Analysis and critique	☐	☐	☐	☐	☐	☐	☐
4. Presentation and delivery	☐	☐	☐	☐	☐	☐	☐
5. Answering questions	☐	☐	☐	☐	☐	☐	☐
6. Quality of educational content	☐	☐	☐	☐	☐	☐	☐
7. Global rating	☐	☐	☐	☐	☐	☐	☐

8. Based on this assessment, how would you rate the Trainee's performance at this stage of training?

Below expectations			satisfactory	better than expected		u/c
☐	☐	☐	☐	☐	☐	☐

Comments:

Assessor's position: Consultant ☐ SASG ☐ Psychologist ☐ Nurse (Band 8 or above) ☐
Other ☐ (Profession: Seniority:)
Assessor's signature......

Please print Assessor's name......

Assessor's Registration number ☐☐☐☐☐☐☐☐   Date:

REFERENCES

Archer, J. C., Norcini, J. and Davies, H. A. (2005). Use of SPRAT for peer review of paediatricians in training. *BMJ*, **330**(7502), 1251–1253.

Archer, J. C., Norcini, J., Southgate, L., Heard, S. and Davies, H. (2008). Mini-PAT (peer assessment tool): a valid component of a national assessment programme in the UK? *Advances in Health Sciences Education*, **13**(2), 181–192.

Babu, K. S., Htike, M. M. and Cleak, V. E. (2009). Workplace-based assessments in Wessex: the first six months. *Psychiatric Bulletin*, **33**, 474–478.

Brittlebank, A. D. (2007). Piloting workplace-based assessment in psychiatry. In *Workplace-Based Assessments in Psychiatry*, ed. D. Bhugra, A. Malik and N. Brown. London: Gaskell, pp. 96–108.

Chisolm, A. and Askham, J. (2006). *What Do You Think of Your Doctor? A Review of Questionnaires for Gathering Patients' Feedback on Their Doctor*. Oxford, UK: Picker Institute.

Crossley, J., Eiser, C. and Davies, H. A. (2005). Children and their parents assessing the doctor–patient interaction: a rating system for doctors' communication skills. *Medical Education*, **39**(8), 820–828.

Davies, H., Archer, J., Southgate, A. and Norcini, J. (2009). Initial evaluation of the first year of the Foundation Assessment Programme. *Medical Education* **43**(1): 74–81.

Department of Health (2003). *Modernising Medical Careers. The Response of the Four UK Health Ministers to the Consultation on Unfinished Business*. London: Department of Health.

Dillner, L. (1993). Senior house officers: the lost tribes. *BMJ*, **307**, 1549–1551.

Downie, R. S. and Charlton, B. (1992). *The Making of a Doctor. Medical Education in Theory and Practice*. Oxford: Oxford University Press.

Fitch, C., Malik, A., Lelliott, P., Bhugra, D. and Andiappan, M. (2008). Assessing psychiatric competencies: what does the literature tell us about methods of workplace-based assessment? *Advances in Psychiatric Treatment*, **14**(2), 122–130.

Holmboe, E. S., Huot, S., Chung, J., Norcini, J. and Hawkins, R. E. (2003). Construct validity of the mini clinical evaluation exercise (miniCEX). *Academic Medicine*, **78**(8), 826–830.

Holmboe, E. S., Hawkins, R. E. and Huot, S. J. (2004). Effects of training in direct observation of medical residents' clinical competence: a randomized trial. *Annals of Internal Medicine*, **140**(11), 874–881.

Julyan, T. E. (2009). Educational supervision and the impact of workplace-based assessments: a survey of psychiatry trainees and their supervisors. *BMC Medical Education*, **9**, 51.

Kogan, J. R., Bellini, L. M. and Shea, J. A. (2003). Feasibility, reliability, and validity of the mini-clinical evaluation exercise (mCEX) in a medicine core clerkship. *Academic Medicine*, **78**(10), S33–S35.

Menon, S., Winston, M. and Sullivan, G. (2009). Workplace-based assessment: survey of psychiatric trainees in Wales. *Psychiatric Bulletin* **33**, 468–474.

Miller, G. (1990). The assessment of clinical skills/competence/performance. *Academic Medicine*, **65**(suppl.), s63–s67.

Norcini, J. J. (2002). The death of the long case? *BMJ*, **324**(7334), 408–409.

Norcini, J. J., Blank, L. L., Arnold, G. K. and Kimball, H. R. (1995). The mini-CEX (clinical evaluation exercise): a preliminary investigation. *Annals of Internal Medicine*, **123**(10), 795–799.

Oyebode, F. (2009). Competence or excellence? Invited commentary on workplace-based assessments in Wessex and Wales. *Psychiatric Bulletin*, **33**, 478–479.

PMETB (2009). *Workplace Based Assessment (WPBA). A Guide for Implementation*. Postgraduate Medical Education and Training Board, Academy of Medical Royal Colleges.

Searle, G. (2007). Evidence-based medicine: case presentation and journal club assessments. In *Workplace-Based Assessments in Psychiatry*, ed. D. Bhugra, A. Malik and N. Brown. London: Gaskell, pp. 76–82.

Sikdar, S. (2010). WPBA or CASC/OSCE: where is it going wrong? *The Psychiatrist*, **34**(1), 72–73.

Smith, J. A. (1995). Semi-structured interviewing and qualitative analysis. In *Rethinking Methods in Psychology*, ed. J. A. Smith, R. Harre, and L. Van Langenhove. London: Sage, pp. 65–92.

Violato, C., Lockyer, J. and Fidler, H. (2003). Multisource feedback: a method of assessing surgical practice. *BMJ*, **326**, 546–548.

Wilkinson, J., Benjamin, A. and Wade, W. (2003). Assessing the performance of doctors in training. *BMJ*, **327**(7416), S91–S92.

Wilkinson, J. R., Crossley, J. G. M., Wragg, A. *et al.* (2008). Implementing workplace-based assessment across the medical specialties in the United Kingdom. *Medical Education*, **42**(4), 364–373.

5

Assessing residents' competencies: challenges to delivery in the developing world – need for innovation and change

Santosh K. Chaturvedi, Prabha S. Chandra and Jagadisha Thirthalli

Editors' introduction

Resource constraints and population pressures in the developing world present unique challenges not only for healthcare delivery but also for postgraduate training. In the past, assessments in postgraduate psychiatric training in the developed countries have relied heavily on examinations that occur infrequently during training. This chapter explores some of the challenges that postgraduate trainees in India need to be trained and assessed for, including the intensity and workload managed by individual clinicians. It also outlines the efforts of one of India's premium psychiatric institutes to assess trainees using both traditional and contemporary methods, in order to enable them to make not only higher-stake decisions at the end of their training, but also to support the trainee's development throughout the duration of training utilizing a range of assessment and feedback strategies.

Introduction

Postgraduate training in psychiatry is more than half a century old in several developing countries. Since the postgraduate psychiatric training followed either the British or the American model, the assessment methods were similar to these models, with local adaptations. The experience from the Indian background is discussed here. Every year, 330 postgraduates train in psychiatry in India, 185 for an MD (Doctor of Medicine) in Psychiatry, 113 for a DPM (Diploma in Psychiatry) and 32 for a DNB (Diplomate of the National Board) in Psychiatry (http://mciindia.org/; http://www.natboard.edu.in/).

This chapter starts by describing the aims and objectives of a postgraduate course and the various assessment methods that have been formally stipulated for

Workplace-Based Assessments in Psychiatric Training, ed. Dinesh Bhugra and Amit Malik. Published by Cambridge University Press. © Cambridge University Press 2011.

postgraduate psychiatric training and are required by the Medical Council of India. It then discusses how far the current assessment methods practised in India are useful in assessing the various competencies that are part of the curriculum. Next, we describe innovative methods of workplace-based assessments that have been used at a leading centre for postgraduate training, and discuss their usefulness in assessment. We also describe the levels of acceptance by trainees of these newer assessment methods. Finally, we make recommendations on the various workplace-based assessments that can be incorporated as part of the overall assessment of psychiatry trainees. Indian literature on postgraduate psychiatric training has also been reviewed briefly.

Workplace-based assessment in developing countries needs to be discussed in light of the workload and duties of the trainees. Clinical services in all teaching hospitals are provided mainly by the postgraduate trainees (also called resident doctors or junior doctors). The healthcare delivery system is unique in that it provides services to all who approach the service, promptly, and on the same day. The training, naturally, also focuses on developing skills to provide prompt services to a large (and unpredictable) number of users. Such a healthcare delivery system is markedly different from that in developed countries, where patients are seen by appointments for fixed periods of time. In an outpatient clinic, patients requiring primary care (walk-in patients), secondary care and tertiary care (specialized services) are all seen by resident doctors at the same time. The services of the trainee doctors are supervised directly by the postgraduate qualified senior residents or by faculty or consultant psychiatrists. In a way, assessment and feedback are continual and form part and parcel of clinical communications between the trainees and the trainers.

Postgraduate psychiatry training in India

There are three types of postgraduate course in India – the MD in Psychiatry or Psychological Medicine (185 places), the Diploma in Psychiatry or Psychological Medicine (DPM, 113 places) and the DNB by the National Board of Examinations (32 places). There are essentially three types of hospital or institutional setting where such training is carried out – mental hospitals that have been reformed and transformed into psychiatric institutes (MD, DPM), general hospital psychiatric units (MD, DPM, DNB) and psychiatric nursing homes (small hospitals offering inpatient and outpatient services) (DNB). The postgraduate training is carried out by 101 centres offering MD, 53 centres offering training in DPM and another 22 centres providing the DNB in psychiatry. Thirteen mental hospital settings converted to teaching institutes provide postgraduate psychiatric training. The mainstay of postgraduate psychiatric training is in the general hospital psychiatric units (Kulhara, 1984). The milestones of psychiatric education at postgraduate level over the last half a century have been described by Agarwal and Katiyar (2004).

The Medical Council of India has laid the following guidelines for postgraduate medical education in India for all specialties (http://mciindia.org/):

1. Postgraduate Medical Education in broad specialties shall be of three years' duration in the case of a degree course and two years in the case of a diploma course after MBBS.
2. The postgraduate curriculum shall be competency-based.
3. Learning in a postgraduate programme shall be essentially autonomous and self-directed.
4. A combination of both formative and summative assessment is vital for the successful completion of the postgraduate programme.
5. A modular approach to the course curriculum is essential for achieving a systematic exposure to the various sub-specialties concerned with a discipline.
6. The training of postgraduate students shall involve learning experience 'derived from' or 'targeted to' the needs of the community. It shall, therefore, be necessary to expose the students to community-based activities.

(Medical Council of India, 2000)

As can be seen from the above guidelines, the importance of formative and summative assessments has been delineated and emphasized. Also emphasized is the fact that the training should focus on the needs of the community. The above guidelines are not very different from those laid down by the National Board of Examinations (http://www.natboard.edu.in/). The Medical Council of India also spells out certain goals and general objectives of the postgraduate medical education programme to be observed by postgraduate teaching institutions. These are as follows:

At the end of the postgraduate training in the discipline concerned, the student shall be able to:

1. Recognize the importance to the concerned specialty in the context of the health needs of the community and the national priorities in the health section.
2. Practice the specialty concerned ethically and in step with the principles of primary healthcare.
3. Demonstrate sufficient understanding of the basic sciences relevant to the concerned specialty.
4. Identify social, economic, environmental, biological and emotional determinants of health in a given case, and take them into account while planning therapeutic, rehabilitative, preventive and primitive measure/strategies.
5. Diagnose and manage majority of the conditions in the specialty concerned on the basis of clinical assessment, and appropriately selected and conducted investigations.
6. Plan and advise measures for the prevention and rehabilitation of patients suffering from disease and disability related to the specialty.
7. Demonstrate skills in documentation of individual case details as well as morbidity and mortality rate relevant to the assigned situation.
8. Demonstrate empathy and humane approach towards patients and their families and exhibit interpersonal behaviour in accordance with the societal norms and expectations.
9. Play the assigned role in the implementation of national health programme, effectively and responsibly.
10. Organize and supervise the chosen/assigned healthcare services demonstrating adequate managerial skills in the clinic/hospital or the field situation.

11. Develop skills as a self-directed learner, recognize continuing education needs; select and use appropriate learning resources.
12. Demonstrate competence in basic concepts of research methodology and epidemiology, and be able to critically analyze relevant published research literature.
13. Develop skills in using educational methods and techniques as applicable to the teaching of medical/nursing students, general physicians and paramedical health workers.
14. Function as an effective leader of a health team engaged in healthcare, research or training.

(Medical Council of India, 2000)

The major components of the postgraduate curriculum are:

- Theoretical knowledge,
- Practical and clinical skills,
- Thesis skills,
- Attitudes, including communication skills,
- Training in research methodology.

(Medical Council of India, 2000)

Postgraduate psychiatric training in India has had a chequered history of growth and development. The difficulties and problems, as well as the developments, have been discussed by Kulhara and Chakraborti (2004), Agarwal and Katiyar (2004) and Channabasavanna (1986). Over time, many disparities in postgraduate training courses have been streamlined and followed as strictly as possible by the Medical Council of India and the National Board of Examinations.

Assessment methods required by the Medical Council of India

The assessment methods include one final examination at the end of three years for the MD course and at the end of two years for the Diploma in Psychological Medicine course. While the Council is fairly clear in outlining the competencies and skills that a postgraduate is supposed to attain, no mention is made of formative assessments, even though this forms part of its initial preamble.

The qualifying examination, which usually lasts a whole day, has the following objectives:

- To assess the theoretical and applied knowledge gained by the trainee in the three-year course;
- To assess the ability of the trainee to function as a competent psychiatrist in the areas of identification, evaluation and management of psychiatric disorders.

(Medical Council of India, 2000)

Theory examination

The theory examination presently comprises five written papers of three hours each, which assess neuroanatomy; neurophysiology, including biochemistry and genetics; clinical psychology, including applied sociology; anthropology and statistics; general psychiatry; recent advances in psychiatry and neurology; and general medicine related to psychiatry.

The theory examination consists of essay-type questions and questions requiring answers in the form of short notes; hence standardization across examiners is not easy, and it is also less objective. Multiple-choice questions do not form part of the examinations, though this is suggested by the Medical Council of India.

Clinical examination

This includes one long case assessment in psychiatry, one long case assessment in neurology and one short case assessment in psychiatry. Some centres keep a 'spotter', while at least one institute examines the trainee on the long-term management of a few clinical cases. This clinical examination is aimed at eliciting the knowledge and competence of the candidates for undertaking independent work as specialists or teachers. However, teaching skills are seldom assessed. There are other variations in the conduct of the clinical and practical examinations, and these are discussed by Kuruvilla (1996).

Oral or viva voce examination

The oral examination aims at eliciting the candidate's knowledge of and competence in the subject, investigative procedures, therapeutic techniques and other aspects of psychiatry, including the scope of all the theory papers. EEGs, radiographic images and results of psychological tests are used during examinations at some centres.

The MD thesis

An important aspect of training and assessment in psychiatry (or any postgraduate MD course in India) is the thesis. The thesis assesses the trainee's ability to formulate research questions and design a simple study. It also helps in training in usage of common scales, analyzing data and critically examining the results.

For many years, the role of a dissertation or thesis was not clear and not followed uniformly. Some institutions expect those taking a diploma to prepare a thesis as well, while some are happy with a published research paper (Wig, 1988). The philosophy behind such research and its controversial viewpoints has been discussed by Wig (1988). Currently, the MCI and NBE insist on a thesis for all MD and DNB candidates; however, the policy for Diploma students varies in different universities.

The thesis is examined by a minimum of three examiners – one internal (the candidate's guide) and two external examiners who need not necessarily be the examiners for the theory and clinical examinations. Acceptance of the thesis by at least two examiners is a precondition for the candidate to appear for the final examination.

Caveats to current assessment methods

The relationship between training goals and assessment

As can be seen from this description, there is a discrepancy between the recommended training and the nature of the assessment that decides whether the trainee passes or fails. While being quite rigorous in terms of its objectives in relation to knowledge and competencies, using a one-day clinical examination to test a trainee is probably not the best method and the reliability and validity of such a method have hardly ever been tested. However, this method is used in most training centres across the world, and also for other clinical subjects other than psychiatry.

Standardization

The case studies for each candidate are selected by the internal and external examiner based on the complexity of the case and its opportunity to test the trainee. However, each trainee gets a different case and therein lies the absence of uniformity and standardization. As the cases are different, the nature of questions asked and issues discussed are different for each candidate. The trainee needs to score at least 50% to be able to pass the examination.

The short case studies are also different for each trainee and the tasks are varied – they may range from making a cognitive assessment to diagnosing cases of psychopathology, such as delusions. As real patients are used for the examination instead of standardized or simulated patients, the ethical issues of patients being made to repeat the same history and participating in assessments become a problem. On the other hand, conducting examinations using simulated patients is far from reality, and this issue has been much debated. There is also the question of using the most cost-effective methods in a resource constrained setting.

The viva voce examination is, however, simpler and gives more opportunity for standardization and objectivity. Trainees are asked a series of questions on various topics by the examiners and an attempt is made to cover areas such as psychotherapy, clinical psychology, sexual medicine, national programmes – to name a few. There is a breadth of coverage; however, this is predominantly knowledge-based.

There is little opportunity in the pattern of examinations for skills assessment. Though in some centres the candidates are asked to interview the patient in front of the examiners, this is based on individual preferences of examiners rather than being a uniform practice.

Advantages of current assessment methods

1. They are elaborate – there are long and short case studies, a neurology case study, assessments of imaging, EEG and psychometry, and a viva voce examination. Long case studies generally consist of a diagnostic or management problem.
2. The long case assessment can be used to assess diagnostic abilities, history taking and eliciting findings. It also gives opportunity to assess approaches to management and whether the trainee is able to discuss both pharmacological and psychosocial methods of management.

Disadvantages of current assessment methods

1. Lacks standardization – so one trainee may be examined on a psychotic disorder, while another trainee may be examined on a personality disorder.
2. It lacks objectivity – no guidelines are given for marking or ranking.
3. It is highly knowledge-based.
4. It is not formative or summative (as the Council would like it to be).

Recommendations for the improvement of assessment methods

Several recommendations have been made by medical educationists in India. They have emphasized a need to rationalize the examination system by giving due emphasis to the 'formative' or internal assessment, introducing logbooks, and supplementing the traditional long and short case examinations with more valid and reliable instruments for the assessment of clinical skills, such as an objective structured clinical examination (OSCE). They recommend that the assessment should predominantly be based on the core curriculum and should be criterion referenced, i.e., the performance of students should be assessed against a standard criterion and not just in comparison with others. The concept of a criterion reference test implies that there is a corpus of knowledge or a standard of skills that the student must possess in order to qualify. In practice, most of the examinations in medicine are norm-referenced or peer-referenced because no clear criteria are laid down beforehand (Sood and Adkoli, 2000).

Medical educationists have emphasized that continual assessment, both formative and summative, is now the norm, with the objective of ensuring clinical competence (Lindsell, 2008). Schuwirth (2004) uses the useful analogy of seeing assessment as a measurement of medical competence and then regarding examinations as diagnostic tools for 'medical incompetence'. As with all diagnostics, examinations have false positive and false negative results with the result that some competent trainees fail while some incompetent ones may pass. These errors need to be minimized as much as possible, as their consequences are serious.

This is where the role of workplace-based assessments becomes important. The periodically summated information about a trainee's performance obtained in these assessments can feed into the formal summative assessments that determine the progress of a trainee from one year to another, culminating eventually into a final assessment as per the requirements of the Medical Council. Ideally, such decisions require a triangulation of evidence, i.e., information from a variety of different sources, to be reliable and meaningful. This means that information from workplace-based assessments, consultant and team feedback, examination results, evaluation of teaching skills, evaluation of research skills, reports from educational supervisors and even patient feedback (or at least some of these) need to be compiled to obtain a reliable assessment.

Internal assessments

Some universities and departments have provisions for internal assessment based on day-to-day clinical work and academic performance. Some use a global rating, while others use a detailed scoring method. The internal assessment scores help in deciding on the passing or failing of a candidate or for deciding the 'topper', i.e., the person scoring maximum marks who stands in first place.

Some innovations in assessment and feedback methods at NIMHANS

The National Institute of Mental Health and Neurosciences (NIMHANS) is a premier institution for postgraduate training in psychiatry and allied behavioural sciences. The first postgraduate training course in psychiatry was started here, in the erstwhile All India Institute of Mental Health, in 1954. Every year, 24 postgraduates are selected for the course following a competitive entrance examination. The MD course runs for three years, while the Diploma course is for two years. At any given time there are nearly 70 trainees in the institute. This necessitates a planned and well-thought-out training programme, adequate supervision methods and periodic feedback. Each trainee (resident) enters the junior residency scheme. An important component of residency is learning while doing rather than focusing only on passive learning methods. Residents are given various clinical postings, including adult psychiatry, child and adolescent psychiatry, consultation liaison, neurology, addiction services, general medicine, community, rehabilitation, behaviour therapy and family therapy. To enhance motivation, contribute to trainer-initiated learning and ensure adequate feedback and assessment, new and creative methods have been evolved in addition to the MCI stipulations. Some of the methods of ongoing assessment and feedback are described here.

Supervision methods

As they rotate through each clinical unit, all trainees are supervised by the unit consultant and senior resident.

Clinical supervision

All cases in the outpatient, inpatient and emergency wards are discussed on a daily basis with a consultant and senior resident. Supervision is also provided by consultants from other disciplines (clinical psychology, social work, neurology) on a case-by-case basis.

Academic supervision

Academic teaching occurs in a group as well as individually. All academic presentations in the unit and the department are supervised by a consultant.

Teaching methods

Seminars, journal clubs and case conferences

These activities happen once every week at the departmental level. These are attended by the faculty, senior and junior residents of the department. Topics for the seminars are chosen from among those suggested by the consultants. These would include a wide range of topics, such as clinical issues, biological psychiatry, psychopathology or psychopharmacology. Each MD course resident has the opportunity of presenting two or three seminars through their course; diploma residents present one or two seminars. The presenter receives active assistance from the chairperson in preparing the presentation. A presentation of about 25–30 minutes is followed by a floor discussion of approximately equal duration, wherein trainees and teachers would discuss the issues raised in the presentation.

For case conferences, each clinical unit chooses an interesting or challenging case to be presented by one of the residents working in the unit. It is chaired by a consultant from a different unit – the resident discusses the case with the consultant in advance. Occasionally, the trainees make brief presentations about literature regarding issues of interest pertaining to the case after the case discussion.

The aim of journal clubs is to familiarize the students with research methodology in psychiatry, with the objectives of enabling them to evaluate research papers critically and to plan simple research projects. At the beginning of every academic year, consultants conduct didactic and workshop-like presentations introducing the students to certain broad areas in psychiatric research, including epidemiology, genetics, clinical trials, qualitative research, systematic reviews, imaging and other biological enquiries. A senior (second- or third-year resident) trainee would present a paper pertaining to the research area covered in the previous week. This series is followed by having the trainees choose articles from leading psychiatry journals and present their critical evaluations of them. These are chaired by consultants, who guide the students in highlighting critical points and discussing their implications. The trainees present the papers for about 15–20 minutes, followed by floor discussion of the article by students and teachers. This is followed by presentation of the presenters' critical evaluation of the paper.

Small-group tutorials on psychopathology and classificatory systems
These activities happen at the unit level, which is a smaller group. Each unit has a weekly case conference chaired by a consultant, and generally attended by the trainees and trainers from the multi-disciplinary team, from psychiatry, psychiatric social work, clinical psychology and psychiatric nursing. Residents and trainees from other specialties take turns to present interesting or challenging cases – trainees from each specialty highlight issues related to their specialty. Topics, generally of clinical interest, are discussed at weekly unit-level seminars or topic discussions. In general, all adult psychiatry units have discussions on psychopathology, basic psychopharmacology, and diagnosis and classification of psychiatric disorders in the initial six months. Units differ in the way they conduct these topic discussions: while some units have a trainee present the topic briefly and have discussions at the end of it, others use group discussions conducted by a moderator, usually a senior resident or a consultant.

A variety of other teaching methods used include debates, quizzes, book reviews, role plays, objective structured clinical examinations (OSCEs) and communication-skills exercises. Feedback is invariably given to the presenters.

Teaching is usually done in groups with peer review and in a multi-disciplinary team. Both didactic and interactive methods are used. Informal teaching as part of case discussions and ward rounds also form an integral part of training.

Rating of and feedback from seminars and journal clubs

The score sheets for rating seminars and journal-club presentations used in NIMHANS are shown in Appendices 5.2 and 5.1, respectively. Each student has about three or four weeks to prepare for each seminar or journal-club presentation. Students are expected to discuss the overall format of presentation with the chairperson and prepare presentation material and handouts in consultation with the chairperson. The score sheets are designed to assess the presentation comprehensively – they assess the content and effectiveness of the presentation and the student's critical evaluation of the subject of the presentation. The presentations are assessed on a scale of 0 to 100. There are 10 domains covering the content, delivery style and depth of understanding of the subject of the presentation. Each domain is scored on a scale from 0 to 10. The first nine domains are evaluated by an average of three or four consultants (but at least two), excluding the chairperson. The chairperson evaluates the trainee's efforts, innovativeness and quality of discussion on a scale of 0–10, for the last domain. At the end of the academic year, the five best seminars and journal-club presentations are awarded with certificates. We have recently concluded an analysis of the previous year's journal-club evaluations – 20 students' journal-club presentations were evaluated. There was high inter-rater reliability across independent assessors for each candidate – intraclass correlation coefficient was 0.73 ($p = 0.004$).

Ethics in clinical care and research

Seminars and workshops related to ethics in psychiatric research are held as part of the training, and students are regularly taught to consider the following:

1. Academic honesty, including acknowledging sources from which material is taken for assignments or seminars;
2. Confidentiality with patients and relatives;
3. Consent procedures;
4. Rational use of patient and institutional resources for patient care;
5. Issues related to conflict of interest;
6. Sensitivity to differences caused by sex or culture.

Modular programmes

This series focuses on basic aspects of clinical psychiatry. The purpose is to encourage students to keep abreast of theoretical aspects of psychiatry on a regular basis. Each module would last three months. An outline of the suggested topics in the area and a list of key references would be provided to the trainees by the coordinator. While faculty members would be requested to give lectures on important topics, the emphasis will be on the trainees to take the initiative to equip themselves with the necessary information in the area concerned. At the end of three months there is a formal written evaluation.

Skill-based teaching and assessment

Adapting the OSCE to become OSCAF – objective structured assessment and feedback

The objective structured clinical examination (OSCE) is commonly used for the assessment of psychiatry trainees but has been used less for teaching. We adapted the OSCE method for postgraduate psychiatry training at our centre. The adapted method was called the objective structured clinical assessment with feedback (OSCAF) (Chandra *et al.*, 2009). The adaptation included several steps: modifying existing OSCE patterns for language and cultural appropriateness, using supervised role playing instead of standardized or simulated patients and developing an assessment method (14-item checklist) that would generate feedback. This exercise was conducted in front of a group of multi-disciplinary peers and supervisors.

Clinical scenarios were selected and adapted after consultation between three psychiatric trainers. These clinical scenarios were then assessed for suitability in relation to content, timing and adaptability to role playing, and used for the study. The case scenarios were chosen to cover a wide spectrum of subjects. Some of them included assessment of psychopathology (depression, thought disorder, suicidal ideation, insight); cognitive function assessments; different clinical conditions, such as substance use, eating disorders, sleep disorders; and different communication and interviewing challenges (education about clozapine, educating a family member about schizophrenia, discussing compliance, breaking bad news). The case scenarios were based on commonly encountered situations in the inpatient, outpatient and emergency settings. Some OSCEs, such as assessing sexual problems, were not selected because of cultural problems in role playing certain topics in front of a peer group.

The 14-item checklist was used to analyze the performance, assessing common elements of any patient-related interaction in 34 different tasks, and the assessments indicated less-than-satisfactory (<75%) performances in the following areas: assuring confidentiality (73.5%), assessing comfort (62%), summarizing (60%), closure (62%) and checking whether the 'patient' had understood what was being communicated (42%). Based on the nature of clinical situations, performances in some specific and difficult OSCAF situations were found to be inadequate and indicated a need for further training. Breaking bad news had the least satisfactory score, followed by assessing delusions, suicidal intent and family history. Assessments of sleep disorders, hypochondriasis, frontal lobe functions, akathisia, compliance, personal history and suitability for behaviour therapy produced the most satisfactory scores.

The results of the debriefing sessions with the trainees indicated that they considered this a useful learning experience. Some reported initial anxiety; however, they felt that the nature of feedback, which was non-judgemental, specific and constructive, helped them. The trainees who simulated patients stated that they were able to empathize with their patients better after having been 'in their shoes' for a short time. The faculty members felt satisfied with the objectivity of ratings and standardization of tasks, which helped them in giving constructive feedback. They also felt that more micro-level teaching was possible, and that emphasis could be laid both on the process and content of the interview. However, different OSCAF situations may require different skills, apart from the 14 skills that were common to all situations. Not being able to assess more specific task-based issues was considered a limitation (Chandra *et al.*, 2009).

Emergency psychiatry

Teaching and assessment in emergency psychiatry is done mainly through workshops held on two afternoons for all first-year residents. A small-group format of teaching is used with case vignettes of different emergency psychiatry situations, such as managing violence, catatonia, acute psychosis, lithium toxicity, suicidality and child psychiatry emergencies.

The workshops follow a skill- and knowledge-based approach. While formal assessments are not made, ongoing assessment and feedback are provided by the senior residents to the trainees on their ability to handle and make appropriate referrals in psychiatric emergencies.

Ongoing assessment and feedback

At the end of each unit posting of three months, trainees are evaluated formally through a variety of methods, which may include a written test (commonly, multiple-choice questions or questions requiring brief answers) or a case discussion (see Appendices 5.3 and 5.4).

Individual feedback is given to each trainee at the end of each posting on both strengths and weaknesses. This includes feedback on punctuality, clinical competence, taking responsibility, decision-making and academic participation. An assessment of the achievement of (skill- and knowledge-based) learning objectives mutually defined at the beginning of the posting is given. Trainees' stress and mental health are also addressed as part of the feedback.

All consultants and senior residents who have trained the trainee are present at the feedback session. In addition to psychiatry consultants, those from clinical psychology and psychiatric social work also provide feedback. Trainees are also encouraged to rate their own performance and the training received at the end of each posting. Internal examinations are conducted in psychology and basic neurosciences at the end of these lecture series.

Thus a trainee on average receives at least ten sessions of feedback or assessment during the course.

Thesis evaluation

The thesis protocol is evaluated by a referee from the department for research and ethical issues. It is then presented to the faculty and student body of the department for further refinement. A protocol thus finalized by the student with these guides is then submitted to the institutional ethics committee for review. Following the completion of the thesis, the results are presented to the department and suggestions for further analysis and discussion are incorporated in the thesis. The thesis is then sent to experts from other centres for external evaluation.

The logbook

Residents are required to keep a comprehensive record of details of their training schedule during their postgraduate tenure, in the form of a logbook. Entries regarding various training activities, unit-level assessments and departmental programmes have to be authenticated by the faculty coordinator concerned. The residents have to maintain the records in duplicate: one copy is to be submitted to the department prior to the final examinations and the other is retained for personal use.

Supervision and feedback on professional issues

Psychiatry is an art as well as a science and one needs to have varying degrees of sensitivity towards several issues while dealing with patients, their families and team members. One also has to be conscious of one's attitude and maintain ethical standards.

Formal and informal feedback is provided to residents about the following issues related to professionalism – manner, attire and attitude, sensitivity towards cultural and sexual differences, boundaries with patients and their relatives, confidentiality and privacy, relationship with pharmaceuticals, relationship with other members of the multi-disciplinary team, and maintaining documentation and progress notes.

Psychotherapy training and assessment

The structured programme started as training in brief dynamic therapy but, over the years, has expanded to include cognitive behavioural and supportive techniques, thus becoming more eclectic in its scope and approach. Faculty members opt to be supervisors. Each supervisor has a trainee group consisting of four to eight residents. The group meets once a week for the entire period of residency.

The training programme starts with a six-session workshop series on interview and communication skills. This is followed by tutorial sessions on basic tenets of dynamic therapy. Thereafter, the trainee therapists take up clients for therapy. Clients are drawn from the outpatient and inpatient services, and across clinical units. Therapy processes and materials are presented in group supervisory sessions. Trainees are encouraged to see a variety of clinical diagnoses and psychosocial contexts.

Diploma trainees (two-year residency) are expected to complete 50 hours of supervised therapy and MD trainees (three-year residency), 75 hours over the residency and training period. The therapy processes are recorded in prescribed session-reporting forms. Over the training period, trainee therapists may see four to ten clients for completed therapy work.

One completed therapy record is submitted for assessment at the end of the programme. This submission includes a detailed process-oriented pro-forma, all the session-reporting forms and a dynamic formulation. The overall assessment is based on the quality of the submission, a presentation based on this and a viva voce. This is conducted by supervisors other than the therapy supervisor of the trainee. In addition, the individual supervisors rate their trainees on adherence to the programme and quality of engagement.

Research on postgraduate psychiatric training and assessment

Not many studies have been published that focus on postgraduate training or assessments. An interesting study 30 years back compared multiple-choice-type questions (MCQs) with tests requiring essay-type answers and short answers (short notes) and found that MCQs correlated poorly with academic competence and competence as a psychiatrist, whereas tests requiring essay-type answers were a better judge of academic competence (Gopinath and Kaliaperumal, 1979). Also published from Indian backgrounds are surveys on facilities for postgraduate training (Kulhara, 1985), and trainees and trainers' viewpoints on training needs and activities (Murthy *et al.*, 1996). Other experienced teachers have discussed the need for a common minimum programme for postgraduate training (Kuruvilla, 1996), suggested modifications for uniform training and assessments (Channabasavanna, 1986), and the teaching of research as a necessary psychiatric skill (Wig, 1988). The recent findings related to use of OSCE and OSCAF (Chandra *et al.*, 2009) have opened doors for standardized, structured and formal workplace-based assessments.

Postgraduate training in some other developing countries

The training programmes vary in duration and content, for example Afghanistan has a three-month diploma while Bangladesh has a $3\frac{1}{2}$-year fellowship programme, a two-year MPhil in psychiatry and a three-year MD psychiatry course (Mullick, 2007). Thailand has a three-year course, with examinations after every year (sometimes after six months) including multiple-choice questions, modified essay and short essay questions, clinical and oral examinations with different pass marks (Udomratn, 2007). Assessment methods in Ethiopia have been described by Hanlon *et al.* (2006), wherein formal assessments included multiple-choice questions, essay questions and mock examinations.

Conclusions – how can we improve and standardize workplace-based assessments?

Kulhara and Chakraborti (2004) suggested continuous monitoring of psychiatric postgraduate training in the form of audits, surveys and feedback from students, to maintain standards as well as enhance quality of teaching and training. Kulhara and Avasthi (2007) also point out a lack of competence-based assessment in the curriculum.

Mendis *et al.* (2004), in an editorial on the topic, emphasized that although the numbers of postgraduates in South Asia have increased, the satisfaction over the numbers completing postgraduate education conceals the challenges facing the region. They emphasize the lack of an appraisal-based approach to training and point out that the selection of assessment tools is not governed by modern educational theory. For example, examinations rely on outmoded assessments, such as essays and long case studies. Training in research, ethical issues, concepts of teamwork and management is variable and not assessed formally as part of training. They also discuss the lack of uniform accreditation methods and the absence of external reviews or internal quality controls of the training and assessment methods. On the other hand, Agarwal and Katiyar (2004) noted that in some centres across the country, the quality of education imparted is near world-class level. They further draw attention to the fact that psychiatry education, training and practice do not require the import and use of expensive equipment or other paraphernalia, rather they have to rely on the judicious use of existing resources.

With this background, it appears that there is a need for a major overhaul in the methods of assessment that reflect current advances in training methods, which could be locally or indigenously developed. Some of the innovations that are currently being used at the Department of Psychiatry at NIMHANS in relation to assessment and feedback methods have been described. However, these still do not find a place in the final assessments, as stipulated by the Medical Council of India: although both formative and summative assessments are performed at every stage, these do not count for the final qualifying examination. This limitation needs to rectified and more objective and standardized methods need to be used.

APPENDIX 5.1 GUIDELINES FOR ASSESSMENT OF JOURNAL-CLUB PRESENTATION

Guidelines of Assessment for Journal Club Presentation

Student: Chair:
                                                   Date:

Please rate on a scale of 0 to 10

1	Organization of slides: Readability, formatting and making the figures, tables, etc., audience-friendly (e.g., not using copy-paste-tables, etc)	
2	Time management (ability to organize the presentation within the time limit)	
3	Presentation style - Form (Effective use of AV aids, voice modulation, body language, eye contact with audience, etc)	
4	Presentation style – Content (Efforts to make the paper understandable to the audience: e.g., use of flow-chart, explaining the procedure/technical terms in simple language, etc)	
5	Level of student's understanding of the presented paper	
	Critiquing the paper	
6a	Critiquing methods and analysis	
6b	Critiquing results, discussion and interpretation of results	
6c	Critiquing the paper as a whole (title, abstract, ethical issues, conflict of interest, etc.) and its implications	
7	Answering questions	
8	Chairperson's evaluation (based on originality, independence, quality of discussion with the chair etc.)	

APPENDIX 5.2 SEMINAR ASSESSMENT FORM

SEMINAR Assessment form

Name of the presenter: **Date:**
Chairperson:
Seminar topic:

Please rate each item on a scale of 0 to 10

PRESENTATION	
Completeness (breadth of coverage of topic, referencing)	
Relevance of content to the topic (adhering to topic, avoiding unnecessary detail)	
Organisation of slide material- fonts, readability, format	
Time Management (ability to organize the presentation within time limit)	
Presentation style (clarity, effective use of AV aids, body language, eye contact with audience)	
Creativity in Presentation- use of flow charts, tables, raising questions)	
Handling questions from the audience and chair	
Summarizing and Concluding	
Critical Evaluation of the topic	

HANDOUT   0-10
   1. Content
   2. Layout
   3. Referencing	

CHAIRPERSON'S EVALUATION ON A SCALE OF 0-10 (Based on originality, independence, presentation style and completeness, quality of discussions with the chair)	

Name and Signature of the Assessor:

APPENDIX 5.3 UNIT-LEVEL FEEDBACK FORMS

Unit Feedback form 1

NURSING/PEER RELATED ISSUES
Communication with peers (residents/other trainees) about patients
Multidisciplinary handing of a case
Communicating with Consultants from other disciplines
Communication and clarity about treatment orders to nurses
Discussion about ward behaviors with nurses

PATIENT RELATED
Availability to the patient in times of crisis
Education about treatment & illness to patients in a way that they can Understand
Ensuring Confidentiality
Involving patients and care givers in decision making regarding treatment
Educating Family members and assessing family issues

KNOWLEDGE
Definitions and examples of psychopathology
Dosage of Drugs
Side effects of Drugs
Diagnoses
Differential Diagnosis
Prognostication
Keeping abreast with latest advances
Keeping abreast with recent studies
Reading classic articles and texts in psychiatry

SKILLS
Handling a violent patient
Managing catatonia
Planning specific psychosocial management
Writing a complete prescription
Writing round notes

PARTICIPATION IN TEACHING PROGRAMS
Prior preparation in all teaching programs
Asking questions and raising issues
Answering questions on the topic

OVERALL ATTITUDE
Listening to patients
Recognising limits of professional competence
Making sure that personal beliefs do not prejudice patients' care
Being professional (in manner, appearance and attitude)

Unit Feedback form 2

FEEDBACK FROM THE UNIT IV TO THE TRAINEE

- ❖ Punctuality/time-management
- ❖ Initiative /motivation
- ❖ Openness / accessibility / approachability
- ❖ Communication/linguistic skills
- ❖ Case presentation skills
- ❖ Critical thinking and discussions
- ❖ Interpersonal and social skills
- ❖ Theoretical knowledge
- ❖ Clinical/diagnostic skills
- ❖ Maintaining records/documentation
- ❖ Probity/sincerity

- ❖ *COMPOSITE COMPETENCE/PERFORMNCE*
- ❖ A : Excellent
- ❖ B : Good
- ❖ C : Average
- ❖ D : Satisfactory/ Further Training
- ❖ E : Below Average / Further Training

SUGGESTIONS FOR FURTHER IMPROVEMENT:

APPENDIX 5.4 OSCE FEEDBACK FORMS

OSCE Feedback from Trainers

Date

Topic / subject:

Trainee

1. Introduction	Unsatisfactory	Satisfactory	Good
2. Confidentiality	Unsatisfactory	Satisfactory	Good
3. Consent	Unsatisfactory	Satisfactory	Good
4. Objective	Unsatisfactory	Satisfactory	Good
5. Establishing Rapport	Unsatisfactory	Satisfactory	Good
6. Paraphrasing	Unsatisfactory	Satisfactory	Good
7. Assessing Comfort	Unsatisfactory	Satisfactory	Good
8. Handling unexpected events	Unsatisfactory	Satisfactory	Good
9. Checking for understanding	Unsatisfactory	Satisfactory	Good
10. Summarizing	Unsatisfactory	Satisfactory	Good
11. Closure	Unsatisfactory	Satisfactory	Good

Content

12. Completeness	Unsatisfactory	Satisfactory	Good
13. Clarity	Unsatisfactory	Satisfactory	Good
14. Correctness	Unsatisfactory	Satisfactory	Good
15. Empathy	Unsatisfactory	Satisfactory	Good

Other comments:

OSCE feedback form : From the trainee doing role play.

A.   Comfort in playing the role
      0 - Very uncomfortable
      1 - A little uncomfortable
      2 - Comfortable
B.   Clarity in playing the role-would have
      0 - Required all inputs
      1 - Require some inputs.
      2 - No inputs required
C.   Satisfaction regarding role play
      0 - not satisfied
      1 - somewhat satisfied
      2 - fully satisfied
D.   How do you rate the interview?
      0 - not satisfied
      1 - somewhat satisfied
      2 - fully satisfied
E.   Overall feeling about Role play
      0- Negative
      1- Can't say
      2- Positive
F.   Any measures to do it differently._____ _____

OSCE Feedback from Interviewer

1.   Comfort
               A. with self as interviewer
                      0 - Very uncomfortable
                      1 - A little uncomfortable
                      2 - Comfortable
               B. performing in front of peer group
                      0 - Very uncomfortable
                      1 - A little uncomfortable
                      2 - Comfortable
               C. being evaluated
                      0 - Very uncomfortable
                      1 - A little uncomfortable
                      2 - Comfortable
               D. feedback in a group
                      0 - Very uncomfortable
                      1 - A little uncomfortable
                      2 - Comfortable
2.   Which component of today's OSCE did you feel most helpful?
               A. Interview
               B. Role play
               C. Improved communication
               D. Feedback
3.   Overall rating about interview.
                  0- not satisfied
                  1-somewhat satisfied
                  2-fully satisfied
4.   Any measures to do it differently._____ _____

REFERENCES

Agarwal, A. K. and Katiyar, M. (2004). Postgraduate psychiatric training in India. II. Status of psychiatric education at postgraduate level. In *Mental Health – An Indian Perspective*, ed. S. P. Agarwal. New Delhi: Elsevier, pp. 218–220.

Chandra, P. S., Chaturvedi, S. K. and Desai, G. (2009). Objective standardized clinical assessment with feedback: adapting the objective structured clinical examination for postgraduate psychiatry training in India. *Indian Journal of Medical Sciences*, **63**, 235–243.

Channabasavanna, S. M. (1986). Psychiatric education. *Indian Journal of Psychiatry*, **28**, 261–262.

Gopinath, P. S. and Kaliaperumal, V. G. (1979). Comparative study of different assessment methods for postgraduate training in psychiatry – a preliminary study. *Indian Journal of Psychiatry*, **21**, 153–154.

Hanlon, C., Fekadu, D., Sullivan, D. and Prince, M. (2006). Teaching psychiatry in Ethiopia. *International Psychiatry*, **3**, 43–46.

Kulhara, P. (1984). Postgraduate psychiatric teaching centres: findings of a survey. *Indian Journal of Psychiatry*, **26**, 281–285.

Kulhara, P. (1985). General hospitals in postgraduate psychiatric teaching and research. *Indian Journal of Psychiatry*, **27**, 221–226.

Kulhara, P. and Avasthi, A. (2007). Teaching and training in psychiatry in India: potential benefits of links with the Royal College of Psychiatrists. *International Psychiatry*, **4**, 31–32.

Kulhara, P. and Chakraborti, S. (2004). Postgraduate psychiatric training in India. I. Current status and future directions. In *Mental Health – An Indian Perspective*, ed. S. P. Agarwal. New Delhi: Elsevier, pp. 215–217.

Kuruvilla, K. (1996). A common minimum programme needed in post-graduate training in psychiatry. *Indian Journal of Psychiatry*, **38**, 118–119.

Lindsell, D. (2008). Changes in postgraduate medical education and training in clinical radiology. *Biomedical Imaging and Intervention Journal*, **4**(1), e19.

Medical Council of India (2000). http://mciindia.org/know/rules/rules_pg.htm.

Mendis, L., Adkoli, B. V., Adhikari, R. K., Huq, M. M. and Qureshi, A. F. (2004). Postgraduate medical education in South Asia. *BMJ*, **328**(7443), 779.

Mullick, M. S. I. (2007). Teaching and training in psychiatry and the need for a new generation of psychiatrists in Bangladesh: role of the Royal College of Psychiatrists. *International Psychiatry*, **4**, 29–31.

Murthy, P., Chaturvedi, S. K. and Rao, S. (1996). Learner centred learning or teacher led teaching: a study at a psychiatric centre. *Indian Journal of Psychiatry*, **38**, 133–136.

Schuwirth, L. W. T. (2004). Assessing medical competence: finding the right answers. *The Clinical Teacher*, **1**(1), 14–18.

Sood, R. and Adkoli, B. V. (2000). Medical education in India – problems and prospects. *Journal of the Indian Academy of Clinical Medicine*, **1**(3), 210–212.

Udomratn, P. (2007). The teaching and training of psychiatry in Thailand. *International Psychiatry*, **4**, 41–42.

Wig, N. N. (1988). Teaching of research as a necessary psychiatric skill. *NIMHANS Journal*, **6**, 1–6.

6

In-training assessment: the Danish experience

Charlotte Ringsted

Editors' introduction

Following a report from the Danish National Committee on Postgraduate Education, Denmark was one of the first developed countries to embark on a journey of developing competency-based training in postgraduate medical education. Traditionally there have been no formal summative or formative assessments in postgraduate medical education in Denmark, with the exception of the appraisal between trainees and their tutors. In this chapter, Ringsted gives a cross-specialty account of anaesthesia and internal medicine in child and adolescent psychiatry, detailing how significant centralized efforts were made across these three specialties to adopt an outcome-based training model, structured on the CanMEDS framework. This included validation of the Canadian framework within the Danish context and the development of tailored outcomes and in-training assessments based on individual specialties, characteristics and tasks. Finally, Ringsted describes the generic lessons learnt from the implementation and evaluation of this outcome-based model in Denmark.

Introduction

In-training assessment (ITA) in postgraduate medical education was introduced in Denmark in 2001, after a report from a Danish National Committee of Postgraduate Education, which recommended a number of innovations regarding structure, process and content of the training, including the introduction of outcome-based education and ITA (Ministry of Health, 2000). Following this report, a reform of postgraduate education was initiated in 2003. Until then, there had been no

Workplace-Based Assessments in Psychiatric Training, ed. Dinesh Bhugra and Amit Malik.
Published by Cambridge University Press. © Cambridge University Press 2011.

assessment of postgraduate trainees in Denmark, apart from regular appraisal meetings between trainees and their tutors.

In Denmark, postgraduate training comes under the jurisdiction of the National Board of Health (NBH) and occurs in defined training posts, in which junior doctors serve a specified number of years. This includes an 18-month mandatory internship, a one-year introductory post in a chosen specialty and, finally, a four- or five-year specialty residency. The introductory year serves as a probationary period during which the trainee can demonstrate suitability for full residency training; vice versa, the trainee can discover whether the specialty seems like a good fit. A trainee can choose to have more than one introductory year, which is not automatically tied to the full residency. Trainees must apply in open competition for residencies and are selected according to qualifications, scholarly proficiencies and other merits as well as prior clinical experience. To this end it is obligatory to have satisfactorily completed an introductory year within the specialty applied for. However, there is no tradition of entry or exit specialist exams, and in general there is a resistance towards examinations in Denmark (Karle and Nystrup, 1995).

Supplementing the clinical training at all stages are some specialty-specific mandatory courses organized at a regional or national level. In addition, following the reform of postgraduate education, a number of general courses on topics such as communication skills, teaching skills, management and organization in health-care, and research have become mandatory. These courses are distributed over the entire period of postgraduate education, from internship to the final specialty training years.

Rationale for in-training assessment

As already discussed in Chapter 1, the rationale for in-training assessment in postgraduate medical education is manifold. Briefly, it relates to the nature of postgraduate education, which is work-based rather than school-based (as is the case for undergraduate medical education). In postgraduate education, trainees are part of the workforce and learn through practising in an authentic clinical setting. This is illustrated in Figure 6.1, inspired by Miller's pyramid (Miller, 1990).

In contrast to undergraduate education, postgraduate education involves much more independent action in practice, with the weighting to the higher levels of Miller's pyramid. Accordingly, assessment strategies should target aspects of 'can and does' rather than being confined to testing knowledge, as traditional specialist examinations do. Moreover, assessment strategies in work-based education have the dual purpose of ensuring trainees' progression towards a predefined educational outcome *and* ensuring patient safety or quality of practice during junior doctors' training. In other words, in-training assessment, spread out over the course of the training, can be used to guarantee that trainees *can do* what they are assigned to in clinical practice. Finally, in-training assessment is probably the

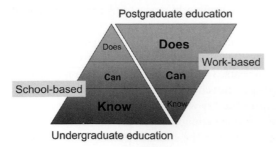

Figure 6.1 Postgraduate work-based education comprises a lot of 'does', action in real practice, as opposed to undergraduate school-based education

only strategy capable of evaluating, in actual practice, outcome-based education in relation to the broad concept of competence (Harden *et al.*, 1999).

Therefore, in Denmark, the National Commission report recommended in-training assessment as an assessment strategy in postgraduate education. Furthermore, as a framework for the broad aspects of clinical competence, they chose to adopt the CanMEDS (see Chapter 10 for more details) and its seven roles: medical expert, communicator, health advocate, collaborator, manager, scholar and professional (Royal College of Physicians and Surgeons of Canada, 2000).

Challenge of introducing in-training assessment

This section describes the challenge of introducing outcome-based education and in-training assessment in postgraduate education related to the Danish context.

Traditionally, postgraduate education has been defined by the number of years in practice and, for some of the surgical specialties, eventually by the number of procedures performed. However, with the introduction of outcome-based education, there was a shift in orientation from quantity and process of training to its quality and outcome. The second challenge was to define learning outcomes based on the CanMEDS framework of seven roles and corresponding aspects of competence. This Canadian framework was initially developed for undergraduate education back in the 1990s for the province of Ontario (Maudsley *et al.*, 2000; Neufeld *et al.*, 1998) and subsequently adapted to postgraduate education in all of Canada (Royal College of Physicians and Surgeons of Canada, 2000). The framework was a result of years of thorough work regarding Canadian society's needs (Frank and Danoff, 2007; Maudsley *et al.*, 2000; Neufeld *et al.*, 1998). Although Canada and Denmark are similar in many ways, there are definitely some differences. Hence, in the Danish context we surveyed the validity of some of the most challenging aspects of competence related to the seven roles (Ringsted *et al.*, 2006a). The response from 3476 Danish doctors, trainees as well as specialists, demonstrated a rather high rating of the importance of the aspects of competence relating to the seven CanMEDS roles; a mean value of 4.2 (SD 0.6) on a scale of 1 to 5. Moreover, this survey revealed that doctors' confidence in the competence framework increased significantly with level of clinical experience. The results also demonstrated some significant differences in ratings of the individual roles in relation to different specialties. Even so, this survey supported content as well as construct validity of the CanMEDS framework in a Danish context.

As in other countries adopting the CanMEDS framework, it was a huge challenge to translate the concept into concrete curricula (Lillevang *et al.*, 2009). The Danish National Board of Health (DNBH) issued some guidelines for the scientific societies of the specialties, who were asked to define outcomes related to the seven roles and propose appropriate in-training assessment strategies. Apart from the guidelines, the DNBH offered consultations from generalists within pedagogies to aid the process of curriculum development. Although the task forces of individual specialist societies were highly motivated and expected that the results would contribute to improve the quality of the specialist education, they also found the process rather frustrating (Lillevang *et al.*, 2009).

Formulating outcomes, in particular related to the non-medical expert roles, was difficult and, in general, the task forces struggled with choosing or designing in-training assessment strategies. To this end, they found neither the guidelines nor the pedagogical experts sufficiently helpful. This most probably reflects the fact that in Denmark the domain of education is based within the humanities, with a qualitative sociologic–pedagogical tradition, as opposed to the situation in many Anglo-American countries, which have a cognitive psychological tradition with a structured, rational approach to education, emphasizing psychometric aspects of assessment (Kuper *et al.*, 2007). Moreover, at the time of the launch of the reform in Denmark, current assessment practice regarding clinical competence did not include either the observation of performance, such as objective structured clinical examinations (OSCEs), or the compilation of documentation of achieved competence in a portfolio, in either undergraduate or postgraduate education. In addition, at that time the international literature regarding in-training assessment was rather sparse. Thus the DNBH and the consulting generalists within pedagogies might themselves have struggled with the paradigm of outcome-based education and in-training assessment.

The resulting curricula first launched in 2004 had a tendency to be overly detailed regarding objectives for the medical expertise role and rather general regarding the other roles. Nevertheless, most specialties revised their curricula in the following years after some initial experience. According to the current DNBH guidelines, clinical supervisors must sign off the entire list of objectives during the course of the training. With the inherent assumption that some sort of assessment lies behind the supervisors' signatures, these documents, together with the collection of certificates of attendance at the mandatory courses, provide the basis for DNBH to grant authorization as specialists. However, some recent studies raise questions as to what extent assessment actually takes place or whether the supervisors' signatures cover a general impression of the trainee (Dehn *et al.*, 2009; Henriksen and Ringsted, 2009). Moreover, these studies indicate that clinical supervisors might conceive that having performed a task is the same as having achieved competence. Therefore, in many cases the supervisor signs off the objectives at the regular appraisal meetings on behalf of the trainee, who has reported having done something without the supervisor actually having observed the performance or seen any other kind of documentation.

This confusion or misinterpretation of the concept of assessment might in part be explained by the fact that historically and culturally postgraduate training followed an apprenticeship model, where access to practice is of paramount importance for professional development. However, unfamiliarity with performance-based assessment in Denmark might be another explanation. Nevertheless, these reports demonstrate a need for initiatives regarding the training of supervisors.

Experiments with constructing in-training assessment programmes

Starting before and continuing during the period when national reform was instigated, we carried out some research and development projects relating to the construction of in-training assessment programmes in three specialties: anaesthesiology; internal medicine; and child and adolescent psychiatry. First in this section is an overview of the process and outcome of the internal rational validation process of designing the in-training assessment programmes and this is followed by an outline of the assessment products related to these programmes, including reports on evaluation studies.

The internal rational validation process

In essence, the process of constructing in-training assessment programmes was the same in all three specialties; a critical review of the literature on professional development and assessment was combined with a participatory design strategy using specialty-specific working groups and studies of the specialty's working practice (Davis *et al.*, 2009; Ringsted *et al.*, 2003a; 2006b). The working groups included trainees at various levels of training and specialists. The process was structured around some basic questions related to developing an in-training assessment programme: why, what, how, when and who. Finally, the strategy included concurrent studies researching parts of the products and evaluating the outcome with the dual purpose of facilitating the development and implementation of the programmes.

The studies of specialty-specific literature and specialties' working practice (including their traditions regarding trainees' professional development) revealed some substantial differences across specialties, shown in Figure 6.2 (Davis *et al.*, 2009; Ringsted, 2004; Ringsted *et al.*, 2003a; 2006b).

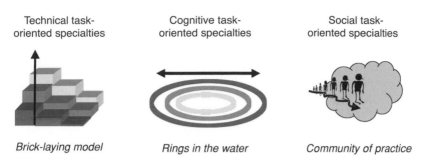

Figure 6.2 The model of trainees' professional development differs according to individual specialties' culture and organization of working practice

Characteristics of anaesthesiology

In anaesthesiology, characterized as a technical task-oriented specialty, novice trainees were typically assigned simple tasks to be fulfilled in rather simple contexts with close supervision. With increasing experience, the trainees tackle gradually more complicated tasks in a variety of complex environments. Typically, a residency training programme consisted of a number of rotations related to the surgical sub-specialties and intensive care units. A brick-laying model could be used to describe the trainees' professional development. The literature and working group discussions revealed that these specialties had a tendency to overemphasize the technical aspects of competence with a weakness regarding cognitive aspects and non-medical expert roles (Ringsted, 2004). In summary, the internal rational validation process indicated a need for a programme that was dispersed over the training course with an emphasis on mastery of basic clinical skills at the beginning and other aspects of competence and reflection on practice at later stages (Ringsted *et al.*, 2003a).

Characteristics of internal medicine

In internal medicine, a cognitive task-oriented specialty, trainees were assigned miscellaneous tasks of varying difficulty (Ringsted *et al.*, 2006b). The expectation was that with increasing levels of experience, the trainees would extend the breadth and depth of task management and take on increasing responsibility in decision-making regarding the management of their patients. The model of professional development thus mirrored ripples in water.

However, trainees' progression and the expectation that they would take on greater responsibility was related to the hierarchical structure of posts based on factors such as their on-call duties, rather than the level of competence that they had actually achieved. Trainees often worked alone and much of the supervision was confined to daily ward conferences. The trainees expressed a need for guidance on how to take a structured approach to their tasks. In particular, this included a need for structure in conducting ward rounds, on acquiring an overview when managing complex cases, being better prepared in dealing with emergency situations and collaborating with other staff.

A preliminary survey of trainees' confidence related to the seven roles demonstrated an irregular pattern of development across training levels, from interns, through first-year trainees, to residents, indicating that different aspects were more important at different times (Davis *et al.*, 2005). Moreover, trainees rated the first-year training as only moderately useful in preparing junior doctors for the seven roles; awarding a score of between 4.8 and 6.6 on a scale of 1 to 10. The lowest-rated role was professionalism, both in terms of trainees' confidence and the training posts' contribution to learning this role. Therefore, the in-training assessment programme in this specialty needed to emphasize a structured approach to managing clinical tasks, connecting medical expertise with the other six roles.

Characteristics of child and adolescent psychiatry

In child and adolescent psychiatry, a social task-oriented specialty, the trainees worked within a dynamic environment with a highly mixed group of professionals, including psychologists, nurses, schoolteachers, childcare and social workers (Davis *et al.*, 2009). The novice trainee's position and contribution to patient management were rather peripheral at the beginning and their legitimacy as team members came from being doctors. With growing experience, the trainees increasingly contributed to patient assessment and management.

However, even as a novice, the trainee could be the only doctor in a team and this caused confusion due to lack of medical professionals as role models within the multi-professional teams. Moreover, as novices, trainees found their medical responsibility within the team overwhelming in cases where they as doctors were supposed to prescribe drugs or take final decisions regarding psychiatric assessment, such as suicide risk. Child and adolescent psychiatry had a strong tradition of remote supervision, although these supervision meetings between trainee and supervisor were rather unstructured. Therefore, in this specialty working groups asked for a programme that could support trainees' preparation for tasks they would be expected to fulfil as doctors, ensure acquisition of psychiatric-specific knowledge and skills, help in clarifying trainees' roles and professional identities within the team, and finally add some structure to meetings with the supervisors.

Purpose, content, format and programming of in-training assessment

The answers to the basic question 'why' were pretty much the same across all three specialties. The assessment programme should serve the purpose of supporting learning and help to structure training and learning while ensuring that all trainees meet a common standard of competence. In addition, the assessment programme should aim to foster an attitude towards systematic analysis and the development of quality of practice.

Regarding content, the working groups acknowledged that it was impossible to assess everything but could offer a few conclusions. For feasibility reasons, the assessment programmes should be confined to crucial tasks, while at the same time covering objectives related to all aspects of the seven roles. Crucial tasks were either commonly performed or were potentially life-saving procedures. Content, format, and programming of the assessment should be tailored to the needs and characteristics of the individual specialties and should reflect the course of professional development during training. The individual assessment instruments should be sufficiently informative both to assessors and trainees and be relevant to practical clinical situations. Task-specific rather than more general assessment instruments were preferred (Davis et al., 2009; Ringsted, 2004; Ringsted et al., 2003a; 2006b).

The assessment products

The products include in-training assessment programmes aimed for the introductory year in all three specialties and for the following four years' residency in anaesthesiology and child and adolescent psychiatry. An outline of the content, format and programming of the three first year ITA programmes is given in Tables 6.1 to 6.3.

Each assessment programme included a number of assessment points and a competence card was provided for each point.

The competence cards depicted the structure and criteria for the assessment and frequently these cards were task-specific rather than general. Moreover, the competence cards often addressed several roles at a time and aimed at linking theory with practice. One category of assessment format was direct observation of trainees' performance; typically the competence card would comprise a checklist including some questions related to cognitive aspects of the task being assessed or non-medical expert roles (see Table 6.4).

Another category of assessment format is the written reflective report, and the accompanying competence card explains the task and criteria for assessment. These assignments typically target issues of quality or systems aspects of practice and scholarly proficiency by relating practice to scientific literature and evidence (see Table 6.5).

A third category was that of structured discussions with a supervisor (see Table 6.6). Here the variety of competence cards ensured appropriate content coverage.

The programme in anaesthesiology included three longitudinal instruments (Ringsted et al., 2003a). One was an experience logbook, the purpose of which was to ensure that trainees acquired sufficient breadth and volume of experience according to a list of recommended numbers of procedures and tasks undertaken during the training year. The second was a continuous quality-monitoring instrument, Cusum scoring, targeting selected procedures and including specified success criteria. The third was a learning portfolio aimed at stimulating self-directed learning. This instrument also appeared in the internal medicine programme.

All in-training assessment programmes, including the competence cards, were made public on the internet to trainees, supervisors and other clinicians, together with guidelines and instructions on assessment procedures. In practice it was left

Table 6.1 Content, format and programming of in-training assessment in anaesthesiology; first-year training

	What	How	When	Who
1.	Managing airways	Direct observation	Before on-call duty, anaesthesia	Any senior clinician
2.	Testing the anaesthesia machine	Direct observation	Before on-call duty, anaesthesia	Any senior clinician
3.	General anaesthesia, elective patient	Direct observation	Before on-call duty, anaesthesia	Any senior clinician
4.	General anaesthesia, emergency patient	Direct observation	Before on-call duty, anaesthesia	Any senior clinician
5.	Preoperative assessment of patient	Direct observation	Before on-call duty, anaesthesia	Any senior clinician
6.	Advanced CPR	Direct observation	Before on-call duty, anaesthesia	Any senior clinician
7.	Spinal anaesthesia	Direct observation	When applicable	Any senior clinician
8.	Epidural anaesthesia	Direct observation	When applicable	Any senior clinician
9.	Central venous catheter	Direct observation	When applicable	Any senior clinician
10.	Plan for fluid and nutrition, ICU	Direct observation	Before on-call duty, ICU	Any senior clinician
11.	Managing simple ventilator, ICU	Direct observation	Before on-call duty, ICU	Any senior clinician
12.	Managing simple ICU case	Direct observation	Before on-call duty, ICU	Any senior clinician
13.	Quantitative experience	Registration of cases, or procedures	1st, 3rd, 6th, 9th, 11th month	Designated supervisor
14.	Quality of experience, selected procedures	Cusum scoring	1st, 3rd, 6th, 9th, 11th month	Designated supervisor
15.	Self-directed learning	Learning portfolio	1st, 3rd, 6th, 9th, 11th month	Designated supervisor
16.	Patient communication	Written report on a patient survey	After 6th month	Designated supervisor
17.	Teamwork and interpersonal skills	Report from two senior colleagues	After 6th month	Designated supervisor
18.	Managing operation list on call	Report from senior colleague on call	After 6th month	Designated supervisor
19.	Anaesthesia and complicating medical diseases	Written assignment	When applicable	Designated supervisor

Table 6.1 (*cont.*)

	What	How	When	Who
20.	Critical appraisal of patient management plan	Written assignment	When applicable	Designated supervisor
21.	Evidence-based medicine	Written assignment	When applicable	Designated supervisor

Table 6.2 Content, format and programming of in-training assessment in internal medicine; first-year training

	What	How	When	Who
1.	Patient encounter, cardiac problem	Direct observation	Within first 3 months	Any senior clinician
2.	Patient encounter, pulmonary problem	Direct observation	Within first 3 months	Any senior clinician
3.	Review of patient record	Senior colleague reviews the patient and assesses trainee's primary patient record	Within first 3 months	Any senior clinician
4.	Follow-up on a complex patient case	Written reflective report	Between 3rd and 6th month	Any senior clinician
5.	Ward round	Direct observation	Between 3rd and 6th month	Any senior clinician
6.	Presentation of patient problem at ward conference	Direct observation	Between 3rd and 6th month	Designated supervisor
7.	Audit on five patient records according to management of fever, pain, nutrition, physical abilities	Written reflective report	After 6 months	Designated supervisor
8.	Evidence-based medicine	Written assignment	After 6 months	Designated supervisor
9.	Presentation skills	Direct observation	After 6 months	Designated supervisor
10.	Professional development	Learning portfolio	At least three times during the year	Designated supervisor

Table 6.3 Content, format and programming of in-training assessment in child and adolescent psychiatry; first-year training

	What	How	When	Who
1.–6.	Patient encounter (unspecified illness category)	Direct observation or video	Every 2 months	Any senior clinician
7.	Team conference (unspecified illness category)	Direct observation or video	When applicable	Designated supervisor
8.	Autism-spectrum disorders	Case-based discussion	When applicable	Designated supervisor
9.	Conduct disorders	Case-based discussion	When applicable	Designated supervisor
10.	Obsessive–compulsive disorders	Case-based discussion	When applicable	Designated supervisor
11.	Personal disorders	Case-based discussion	When applicable	Designated supervisor
12.	Attention-deficit disorders	Written reflective case analysis	When applicable	Designated supervisor
13.	Affective disorders	Written reflective case analysis	When applicable	Designated supervisor

to the trainees to initiate these assessments. On completion of an assessment, the assessor signed the competence card and the trainee filed this in a portfolio. A designated supervisor helped the trainee in getting started with the line of assessments and kept track of progress at regular appraisal meetings. In the event that a trainee didn't pass an assessment, due remediation was meant to be initiated and the trainee would subsequently be assessed again. However, it was necessary that the trainees eventually passed all assessments included in the entire programme in order to get a certificate. If they didn't reach this during the designated training period, educational authorities would arrange for extra training time in an appropriate post.

Anaesthesiology

In-training assessment programmes in anaesthesiology were nationwide. The first-year ITA programme was introduced in 2001 and a revised version, together with the residency programme, was introduced in 2004. The initial first-year ITA programme included 21 elements spread over the entire year, as illustrated in Figure 6.3 (Ringsted et al., 2003a).

The skills assessments were mandatory for a licence to practice and had to be passed before the trainees were allowed to undertake on-call duties or work without close supervision. Therefore, many skills assessments were placed rather early on in the training year, while assessment of other aspects of competence came later.

Table 6.4 Example of a competence card for assessment of ward-round performance by direct observation

Ward-round	Score 1–5
Introduction and preparation	
Clarify who will be on the team for this ward round. Setting the scene by discussion with the team members	☐
Explore any organizational problems that might influence patient management, such as current and expected patient load, shortage of staff, other	☐
Patient round	
Reviews patient record and charts and gets an overview related to prior investigation and management plan.	☐
Reviews recent investigations, medicine prescriptions, etc., and performs relevant follow-up and adjustments.	☐
Performs an efficient patient consultation and includes staff observations and other relevant information.	☐
Focuses together with the team the medical problems that need further management.	☐
Summarizes management plan together with patient and team. Specifies problems and decisions that need consultation with senior colleague.	☐
Ensures that patient understands and agrees to plans and decisions	☐
Summary, conclusion, and evaluation	
Summarizes the ward round with the team and prioritizes problems and actions	☐
Reviews deals with the team and summarizes information that should be conferred to other staff and colleagues	☐
Evaluates the process of the ward round with the team	☐
Overall assessment of the performance	☐

In the four-year residency programme the emphasis was on complicated tasks and procedures with increasingly complex and critical situations on the agenda. Examples are managing unexpected difficult airways, team conflicts and critical incidents or errors. These aspects of competence were assessed by reflective reports on actual events. Accompanying competence cards indicated a structural approach to the analysis according to issues of medical expertise, systems and organizational aspects, human resources, communication and collaboration. Additionally, management and leadership skills were assessed either by observation or by use of a 360-degree instrument. Finally, both of the ITA programmes launched in 2004

Table 6.5 Example of competence card related to a written assignment in anaesthesiology

Written assignment

This assignment includes:
1. A critical reflection on a patient case according to clinical guidelines and literature
2. An in-depth analysis of a specific problem related to literature and
3. A written report

1. *Critical reflection on patient case*
   Describe the case of a patient who has been in general anaesthesia and relate it to recommendations in the guidelines, literature and textbooks. Analyze the case and describe unexpected issues or complications.

2. *Problem formulation and literature search*
   Define a problem you want to examine further through a literature search. Perform the search, assess and discuss the results of your search relating to the problem. Consider whether your conclusions might influence your own or the department's practice. Present your consideration at the conference.

3. *Report (max. 4 pages), must include*
   Introduction of formulation of problem, criteria for literature search, results of the search, discussion of results, conclusion and implications for practice

Give the report to your supervisor, who will assess it according to the criteria listed below

The report includes:

Clear, concise and sufficient description of patient management	☐
Clear problem formulation and rationale for choice of problem to study further	☐
Precise formulation of criteria for literature search	☐
Rationale for choice of references used to analyze problem	☐
Conclusion regarding literature search	☐
Discussion of results' significance to managing the problem	☐
Conclusion and implications for own or department's practice	☐
Overall assessment	☐

included a general assessment instrument to be used regularly in each rotation or at least every six months. This instrument was related to each of the seven roles and to breadth and volume of experience according to the task and procedure list. The instrument indicated carefully defined expectations regarding outcome for each of the seven roles according to either first-year training level or specialist level.

Table 6.6 Example of a competence card related to case-based discussion between supervisor and trainee in child and adolescent psychiatry

Pervasive developmental delay	
Diagnosis	**Score 1–5**
State a minimum of three essential diagnostic criteria for pervasive developmental delay. Describe and justify which investigations the physician should choose to make the diagnosis.	☐
Describe the age-dependent characteristics that have an influence on the diagnostic criteria	☐
Give three relevant differential diagnostic considerations within this diagnostic group and state which investigations must be undertaken to differentiate them	☐
Give three relevant differential diagnostic considerations outside of this diagnostic group and state which investigations must be undertaken to rule them out	☐
Age variation	
Describe the age-related variations within this diagnostic group by giving theoretical descriptions of the expected findings in a 5-year-old patient, a 10-year-old patient, and a 15-year-old patient	☐
Diagnostic work-up	
Describe the classic diagnostic work-up for two of the sub-diagnoses in this diagnostic group, with reference to the newer relevant literature as well as to which other health professionals it would be important to involve	☐
Written communication on actual patient course to collaborators	
Write a short and relevant report of the background information, formulated in easy-to-read professional language	☐
Give a report of the essential findings in the diagnostic work-up, formulated in easy-to-read professional language	☐
Recommend support and treatment measures	☐
Give prognosis based on the working diagnosis	☐
Overall assessment of discussion and written report of pervasive developmental delay	☐

The preliminary first-year ITA programme has been extensively studied. Initially, consultants' opinions of the content, format and programming were surveyed (Ringsted *et al.*, 2002). Responses from 251 out of 382 consultants (66%) demonstrated a median score of 4 or 5 on a scale of 1 to 5, regarding importance, relevance and sufficiency of content in all the assessments. Interquartile ranges were low, except for 'managing operating list on call' and 'evidence-based

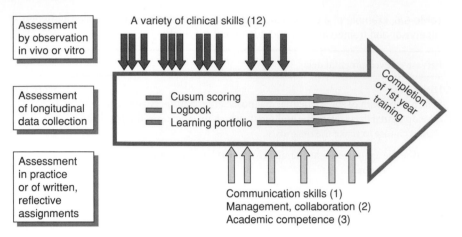

Figure 6.3 An in-training assessment programme for the introduction year in anaesthesiology

medicine assignment', where the 25th percentile was 3, as opposed to 4 or 5 in all other assessments. This meant that problems regarding implementation of these two assessments were foreseen.

A second study consisted of an experimental set-up where consultants were randomly divided into two groups, each using one of the two scoring formats to assess a trainee's performance in four different simulated clinical scenarios on videotape (Ringsted *et al.*, 2003b). In three of the scenarios, the trainee made one serious and one minor mistake. One scoring format was a task-specific checklist and the other was a more global scoring form with broad categories of competence. Results demonstrated that consultants preferred task-specific checklists to the global scoring form. However, inter-rater agreement regarding pass and failure was poor, irrespective of the scoring form used. This finding was attributed to clinicians' leniency as assessors rather than to a lack of vigilance regarding the mistakes. Therefore, although this study confirmed the appropriateness of using task-specific competence cards in the ITA programme, the results also indicated a need for training of clinicians as assessors.

A preliminary study of the implementation and acceptability of the first-year ITA programme was conducted 18 months after the introduction (Ringsted *et al.*, 2003c). Responses from 96% of a total of 26 departments of anaesthesiology showed that 83 out of 100 trainees had been enrolled in the programme. Evaluation from trainees demonstrated that in general the programmes were highly valued in clarifying goals and objectives and emphasizing aspects of competence that would probably not have been covered otherwise. In general, the programme was seen as being of help in structuring training, teaching and learning and fostering learning through studying for the tests and through the feedback on performance. However, the trainees also pointed to problems with assessors being unfamiliar with the concept and content of assessments and difficulties in finding time in a busy clinical workplace. The assessments targeting clinical skills were highly appreciated with median ratings of 7 or 8 on a scale of 1 to 9. Rather unexpectedly, the trainees valued highly the two assessments of organizational and management skills (median 8) and the three written assignments (median 7). In contrast, they had mixed feelings towards the experience log, Cusum scoring and learning portfolio, all having a median rating of 5 with large interquartile ranges. The communication skills assessment was also rated rather poorly (median 5).

In a following qualitative study, we interviewed the users of the ITA programme, programme directors, supervisors and trainees, regarding how the programme worked in practice and what benefits and barriers they perceived (Ringsted *et al.*, 2004a). The results supported the preliminary evaluation data in that all three parties found the programme helpful in structuring training, teaching and learning. The senior clinicians emphasized that they also learned from the programme, especially regarding the broader aspects of competence. The trainees appreciated the coupling of practice to theoretical aspects and all three parties indicated that the programme fostered an academic dialogue in the departments. Moreover, the programme was useful in monitoring trainees' progress and in helping to identify and manage trainees in difficulty.

Respondents emphasized the motivating and meaningful issues of coupling assessment to patient safety and quality of practice, both in terms of using in-training assessment progressively as a licence to work more independently in practice and in the ability of the new format to combine theoretical and practical aspects of clinical training. The data also indicated that the assessment protocol was not always followed as stipulated and in cases where trainees were assessed after they had been performing procedures independently for some time they found the assessment 'a meaningless marking on a sheet of paper'. Similar statements also referred to cases of lenient assessors. Neither trainees nor supervisors found mere documentation of competence important. Instead, respondents indicated that the assessment should include a challenge in order to have an effect on learning. Trainees valued assessments that they learned from even if they didn't pass on the first attempt. Thus both trainees and supervisors found the communication assessment meaningless because trainees only got high ratings from their individual surveys of 25 patients. In summary, analysis of the data revealed three inter-relating factors that influenced the perceived value of ITA: linking assessment to practice; educational benefit; and the attitude and rigour of assessment.

Finally, we aimed to study the effect of the ITA programme by carrying out a national survey of anaesthetists' confidence in managing an array of 155 tasks and procedures covering the entire specialist training curriculum (Ringsted *et al.*, 2004b). The study was a cross-sectional survey of trainees at all levels, before and two years after the introduction of the first-year ITA programme. Responses from 377 trainees out of 531 (71%) in 2001 and from 344 trainees out of 521 (66%) in 2003 showed no significant impact of in-training assessment on confidence levels, either in aspects related to the first-year ITA programme or in other aspects.

In 2004, a revised version of the first-year ITA programme was launched, together with a programme for the four-year residency. The introduction of these two nationwide programmes was supported by a number of courses for assessors (Maling *et al.*, 2007). The courses used the videos from the former study of scoring formats to give training in assessment procedures and to give feedback to the trainee. Evaluation of the course was very positive and the course had a long-lasting effect on participants' knowledge of the assessment procedures. A recent survey demonstrated that the first-year programme has been adequately implemented (Skjelsager *et al.*, 2008).

Internal medicine

The ITA programme in internal medicine for first-year trainees was introduced in 2002 on a regional basis. This programme was less ambitious than that for use in anaesthesiology and included only 10 assessment points (Ringsted *et al.*, 2006b). Included in the programme was a list of the 35 essential conditions or problems that the trainee should learn to manage. The list was meant to guide trainees' self-directed learning plans, which are meant to be discussed at regular meetings with a designated supervisor. This list was constructed from analysis of case-mix data across all hospitals in the capital. Accompanying the programme were some simulation-based courses in emergency medicine and a course on ethics and professionalism.

A couple of evaluation studies were connected to this programme. Firstly, validity of the ward-round assessment was studied (Norgaard *et al.*, 2004). Content validity regarding relevance and comprehensiveness of items on the competence card was surveyed among 295 interns. The results from 238 (81%) respondents showed a general agreement on the relevance and comprehensiveness of the card. Not surprisingly, the items related to medical expertise were rated as being more relevant than items related to interpersonal and organizational skills. The second part of this study concerned the construct validity of assessment using the competence card. Ward-round performance was observed and assessed across four groups of doctors with increasing levels of experience; interns, first-year trainees, residents and consultants. The results demonstrated a significant increase in median checklist score (a scale from 0 to 4) over the four groups, from 1.4 for the most junior doctors to 2.7 for consultants. The reason why even consultants did not attain proficiency scores of level 4 was that all four groups scored relatively poorly in the non-medical expertise aspects. This indicates that all parties, trainees as well as consultants, might benefit from using the competence card to focus on interpersonal and organizational aspects of competence.

Preliminary evaluation of the entire programme with data from 25 first-year trainees demonstrated that the assessment procedures most highly valued were 'ward round', 'presentation at conference', 'evidence-based medicine' and 'oral presentation', with median scores of 7 on a scale from 1 to 9. Assessments related to 'audit of patient records' and 'follow-up on a complex patient case' were moderately valued, achieving a median score of 6.5, and the three patient-encounter assessments were the least valued, with a median score of 5 or 6.

The trainees commented that the ITA programme was of help in structuring learning and training and increasing supervision and feedback on performance. They valued having an overview of what they were supposed to learn and having an explanation of some of the non-medical expert aspects. Some felt that patient-encounter assessments were more relevant to a lower level of training, i.e., internship or senior undergraduate years. Just as in anaesthesiology, the value of assessments was related to the supervisor's enthusiasm. Time constraints were the most frequent concern regarding fulfilment of the programme; in particular, being observed during performance seemed to be problematic.

Because of the concurrent national reform process, the preliminary programme was abandoned in 2004 and various other initiatives took over. In internal medicine there is now a trend towards adopting more general assessment instruments, such as the mini-CEX and 360-degree evaluations (Allerup *et al.*, 2007; Eriksen *et al.*, 2009).

Child and adolescent psychiatry

In child and adolescent psychiatry, the ITA programme for first-year trainees was centred on eight task- or disorder-specific competence cards (Davis *et al.*, 2009). The emphasis was on basic skills and knowledge related to the patient encounter, but non-medical expert roles, such as those of communicator, collaborator, manager and scholar were also addressed, linking practical issues to theory. Over the residency years, the competence cards were increasingly designed to promote clinical reasoning skills related to pertinent aspects of patient care and to encourage evidence-based inquiry and critical review and reflection on practice. Until now, no evaluation studies have been conducted on these programmes.

Lessons learned and perspectives

In summary, experiments of constructing in-training assessment programmes within three different specialties resulted in the following lessons:
1. The overall aim of in-training assessment should be to help structuring learning, teaching and training.
2. ITA should be tailored to specific characteristics of specialties, their tasks and working practice, and combine broad definitions of competence with lists of tasks, procedures and situations that trainees should experience.
3. ITA should be closely linked to quality of practice and, when possible, be used as evidence to support licence for independent practice.
4. Standards of performance can be defined in overall learning outcomes and further detailed in competence cards.

5. ITA programmes should include increasingly more challenging learning objectives and be appropriate to the trainees' level of professional development.
Some of these aspects are further discussed here.

The postgraduate education context is a busy clinical workplace with patient
care being its primary objective. Therefore, both parties – trainees and teachers –
emphasized the practical considerations of implementing ITA programmes in
a manner that helped obtain an overview of the trainee's educational development supported structuring learning and training without the process becoming a
bureaucratic burden. In general, introducing outcome-based education related to
broad aspects of competence and designing corresponding in-training assessments
was a challenge and required a shift in mindset. In principle, the new concept of
outcome-based education should replace the former detailed learning objectives
and quantitative standards in postgraduate training.

Harden's model of outcome-based education portrays three layers, an inner core
of knowledge and skills, a medium level relating to the approach to the tasks, and
finally an outer layer including professionalism (Harden *et al.*, 1999). The concept
of competence relates to the integration of all three layers, just as the CanMEDS
framework relates to an integration of medical expertise with the other six roles
(Frank, 2005).

However, since the introduction of the concept a decade ago, even after all these
years, there has been a tendency for a fragmented perception of the concepts of
competence rather than a holistic view of competence (Huddle and Heudebert,
2007; Zibrowski *et al.*, 2009). The concept of competence is often used interchange-
ably with the concept competency. While the term competence relates to a generic
and holistic meaning referring to an overall capacity, the term competency often
refers to a specific capability or skill (Eraut, 1999). Epstein and Hundert (2002)
define competence as

The habitual and judicious use of communication, knowledge, technical skills, clinical
reasoning, emotions, values, and reflection in daily practice for the benefit of the individual
and the community being served.

This definition emphasizes both the integration of all aspects of competence
and a close link to practice. The challenge, however, lies in applying this concept
in a concrete postgraduate educational context, and in formulating learning goals
and objectives that can guide the trainees' professional development (Norman,
2006).

In our experiments, we chose a highly context-bound approach and tailored the
objectives and accompanying ITA programmes to individual specialties' characteristics and tasks. To help structure training and learning, we combined
qualitative defined outcomes regarding the approach to the tasks and issues of
professional conduct with quantitative lists indicating specific standards corresponding to the breadth and volume of a trainee's experience. In support of
this approach, the literature on the development of expertise emphasizes that
both quantity and quality of experience are equally essential (Ericsson, 2004).

Therefore, abandoning postgraduate traditions of measuring experience and stipulating required number of years in practice might be 'throwing out the baby with the bathwater'.

A central issue in postgraduate education is the trainees' wish for and the culture's expectation of independency and autonomy in managing tasks (Dijksterhuis *et al.*, 2009; Hinchey *et al.*, 2009; Kennedy *et al.*, 2009). This imperative relates to a step-wise mastery-learning model that fits well with some aspects of technical task-oriented specialties. In our experiment with anaesthesiology, this approach was taken from the very beginning of the first-year ITA programme, where evidence from assessments was used as a licence to practice, thereby making a close connection between assessments, patient safety and quality of clinical practice. However, technical task-oriented specialties include many other aspects of competence besides mere technical expertise, and for these a mastery-learning model is not feasible. Moreover, such a model does not make sense in cognitive- and social-oriented specialties. Yet our experience of using ITA focused on structuring the approach to tasks and supporting reflections on the continuous improvement of individual and systems-based aspects of clinical practice. In essence, postgraduate education is a preparation for future learning. In this context, ITA programmes that support both the efficiency and innovative dimension of development of expertise are worth striving for (Schwartz *et al.*, 2005). The structured competence cards in the ITA programmes related to increasingly challenging tasks and both trainees and trainers appreciated that the cards supported learning, in particular in areas not otherwise addressed in the postgraduate medical education. However, assessments that did not include a challenge were less acceptable and were perceived as a meaningless, bureaucratic event.

The Danish system had not previously used assessment in postgraduate education and the ITA approach was chosen over final examinations. The advantage of this choice was an incentive to design elaborate ITA programmes based on a rational internal validation process that included literature study, discussions among users and concurrent research projects. This approach has recently been advocated by international experts in assessment (Dijkstra *et al.*, 2010). There is no doubt that the developmental process has contributed to the implementation of ITA. However, much more research is needed to explore the educational impact of such programmes.

REFERENCES

Allerup, P., Aspegren, K., Ejlersen, E. *et al.* (2007). Use of 360-degree assessment of residents in internal medicine in a Danish setting: a feasibility study. *Medical Teacher*, **29**, 166–170.

Davis, D. J., Skaarup, A. M. and Ringsted, C. (2005). A pilot survey of junior doctors' confidence in tasks related to broad aspects of competence. *Medical Teacher*, **27**, 548–552.

Davis, D. J., Ringsted, C., Bonde, M., Scherpbier, A. and Van Der Vleuten, C. (2009). Using participatory design to develop structured training in child and adolescent psychiatry. *European Child and Adolescent Psychiatry*, **18**, 33–41.

Dehn, P., Nielsen, C. H., Larsen, K. and Bayer, M. (2009). Implementering af speciallægereformens syv roller [Implementing the seven roles of the specialist training reform]. *Ugeskrift for Læger*, **171**, 1580–1584.

Dijksterhuis, M. G. K., Voorhuis, M., Teunissen, P. W. *et al.* (2009). Assessment of competence and progressive independence in postgraduate clinical training. *Medical Education*, **43**, 1156–1165.

Dijkstra, J., Van Der Vleuten, C. P. M. and Schuwirth, L. W. T. (2010). A new framework for designing programmes of assessment. *Advances in Health Sciences Education*, **15**(3), 379–393.

Epstein, R. M. and Hundert, E. M. (2002). Defining and assessing professional competence. *JAMA*, **287**, 226–235.

Eraut, M. (1999). Concepts of competence and their implications. In *Developing Professional Knowledge and Competence.* ed. M. Eraut. London: The Falmer Press, pp. 164–181.

Ericsson, K. A. (2004). Deliberate practice and the acquisition and maintenance of expert performance in medicine and related domains. *Academic Medicine*, **79**, S70–S81.

Eriksen, J. G., Simonsen, D., Bastholt, L. *et al.* (2009). Mini-clinical evaluation exercise til evaluering af kommunikation og samarbejde i ambulatoriet [Mini clinical evaluation exercise as evaluation tool of communicative and cooperative skills in the outpatient clinic]. *Ugeskrift for Læger*, **171**, 1003–1008.

Frank, J. R. (ed.) (2005). *The CanMEDS 2005 Physician Competency Framework. Better Standards. Better Physicians. Better Care.* Ottawa, ON: Royal College of Physicians and Surgeons of Canada.

Frank, J. R. and Danoff, D. (2007). The CanMEDS initiative: implementing an outcomes-based framework of physician competencies. *Medical Teacher*, **29**, 642–647.

Harden, R. M., Crosby, J. R. and Davis, M. H. (1999). *AMEE Guide No.* 14: Outcome-based education Part 1 – an introduction to outcome-based education: a model for the specification of learning outcomes. *Medical Teacher*, **21**, 7–14.

Henriksen, A. H. and Ringsted, C. (2009). Vejlederes holdninger til kompetencevurdering af turnuslæger [Clinical supervisors' perceptions concerning assessment of pre-registration house officers]. *Ugeskrift for Læger*, **171**, 1505–1508.

Hinchey, K. T., Iwata, I., Picchioni, M. and McArdle, P. J. (2009). "I can do patient care on my own": autonomy and the manager role. *Academic Medicine*, **84**, 1516–1521.

Huddle, T. S. and Heudebert, G. R. (2007). Taking apart the art: the risk of anatomising clinical competence. *Academic Medicine*, **82**, 536–541.

Karle, H. and Nystrup, J. (1995). Comprehensive evaluation of specialist training: an alternative to Board examinations in Europe? *Medical Education*, **29**, 308–316.

Kennedy, T. J. T., Regehr, G., Baker, G. R. and Lingard, L. A. (2009). 'It's a cultural expectation . . . ' The pressure on medical trainees to work independently in clinical practice. *Medical Education*, **43**, 645–653.

Kuper, A., Reeves, S., Albert, M. and Hodges, B. D. (2007). Assessment: do we need to broaden our methodological horizons? *Medical Education*, **41**, 1121–1123.

Lillevang, G., Bugge, L., Beck, H., Joost-Rethans, J. and Ringsted, C. (2009). Evaluation of a national process of reforming curricula in postgraduate medical education. *Medical Teacher*, **31**, e260–e266.

Maling, B., Bested, K. M., Skjelsager, K., Østergaard, H. T. and Ringsted, C. (2007). Long-term effect of a course on in-training assessment in postgraduate specialist education. *Medical Teacher*, **29**, 966–971.

Maudsley, R. F., Wilson, D. R., Neufeld, V. R. *et al.* (2000). Educating future physicians for Ontario: Phase II. *Academic Medicine*, **75**, 113–126.

Miller, G. (1990). The assessment of clinical skills/competence/performance. *Academic Medicine*, **65**, S63–S67.

Ministry of Health (2000). *Fremtidens speciallæge. Betænkning fra Speciallægekommissionen* [*The Future Specialist. Report from the Specialist Commission*], Report no 1384. Copenhagen: Statens Information.

Neufeld, V. R., Maudsley, R. H., Pickering, R. J. *et al.* (1998). Educating future physicians for Ontario. *Academic Medicine*, **73**, 1133–1148.

Norgaard, K., Ringsted, C. and Dolmans, D. (2004). Validation of a checklist to assess ward round performance in internal medicine. *Medical Education*, **38**, 700–707.

Norman, G. (2006). Outcomes, objective, and the seductive appeal of simple solutions. *Advances in Health Science Education*, **11**, 217–220.

Ringsted, C. (2004). *In-Training Assessment in a Work-Based Postgraduate Medical Education Context*. Ph.D. thesis, Universitaire Pers Maastricht, the Netherlands: Datawyse.

Ringsted, C., Østergaard, D. and Scherpbier, A. (2002). Consultants' opinion on a new practice-based assessment programme for first-year residents in anaesthesiology. *Acta Anaesthesiologica Scandinavica*, **46**, 1119–1123.

Ringsted, C., Østergaard, D. and Scherpbier, A. (2003a). Embracing the new paradigm of assessment in residency training: an assessment programme for first-year residency training in anaesthesiology. *Medical Teacher*, **25**, 54–62.

Ringsted, C., Østergaard, D., Ravn, L. *et al.* (2003b). A feasibility study comparing checklists and global rating forms to assess resident performance in clinical skills. *Medical Teacher*, **25**, 654–658.

Ringsted, C., Østergaard, D. and Van Der Vleuten, C. P. M. (2003c). Implementation of a formal in-training assessment programme in anaesthesiology and preliminary results of acceptability. *Acta Anaesthesiologica Scandinavica*, **47**, 1196–1203.

Ringsted, C., Henriksen, A. H., Skaarup, A. M. and Van Der Vleuten, C. P. M. (2004a). Educational impact of in-training assessment (ITA) in postgraduate medical education: a qualitative study of an ITA programme in actual practice. *Medical Education*, **38**, 767–777.

Ringsted, C., Pallisgaard, J., Østergaard, D. and Scherpbier, A. (2004b). The effect of in-training assessment on clinical confidence in postgraduate education. *Medical Education*, **38**, 1261–1269.

Ringsted, C., Hansen, T. L., Davis, D. and Scherpbier, A. (2006a). Are some of the challenging aspects of the CanMEDS roles valid outside Canada? *Medical Education*, **40**, 807–815.

Ringsted, C., Skaarup, A. M., Henriksen, A. H. and Davis, D. (2006b). Person-task-context: a model for designing curriculum and in-training assessment in postgraduate education. *Medical Teacher*, **28**, 70–76.

Royal College of Physicians and Surgeons of Canada (2000). CanMEDS 2000: Extract from the CanMEDS 2000 project societal needs working group report. *Medical Teacher*, **22**, 549–554.

Schwartz, D. L., Bransford, J. D. and Sears, D. (2005). Efficiency and innovation in transfer. In *Transfer of Learning From a Modern Multidisciplinary Perspective*, ed. J. Mestre. Greenwich, CT: Information Age Publishing, pp. 1–52.

Skjelsager, K., Malling, B., Bested, K. M. *et al.* (2008). Implementering af nationalt kompetenceprogram i anæstesiologi. [Implementation of a national training assessment programme in anaesthesiology.] *Ugeskrift for Læger*, **170**, 3557–3561.

Zibrowski, E. M., Singh, S. I., Goldszmidt, M. A. *et al.* (2009). The sum of the parts detracts from the intended whole: competencies and in-training assessments. *Medical Education*, **43**, 741–748.

7

The US experience of changing roles

Richard Summers

Editors' introduction

The challenges of making summative decisions using programmes of workplace- or performance-based assessments have been previously rehearsed in literature and elsewhere in this volume. In this chapter, Richard Summers outlines the traditional roles of the various statutory and professional bodies involved in postgraduate psychiatric training in the United States of America. The chapter also describes the systemic changes in regulations and requirements concerning postgraduate assessment at a national level, including the move from external standardized skill-based assessments to local programme-based assessments, which resulted in a transfer of some of the high-stake decision-making to local programme directors rather than a national statutory body. The debates and dilemmas, nationally and locally, that have resulted from this systemic change and the manner in which various stakeholders have responded to it are also summarized. Summers concludes by highlighting the advantages of and challenges posed by this seismic shift in the assessment of psychiatric residents in the United States.

Richard Summers thanks Deborah Cowley, MD, for her advice in preparing this chapter.

Introduction

The time-honoured method for assessing the clinical skills of future psychiatrists in America reflected a tradition of local programme diversity paired with national consensus standards. The system allowed for checks and balances between education and assessment in residency training programmes and an examination administered by the national certifying body, the American Board of Psychiatry and Neurology (ABPN). Recently, a variety of forces have combined to reconfigure

Workplace-Based Assessments in Psychiatric Training, ed. Dinesh Bhugra and Amit Malik.
Published by Cambridge University Press. © Cambridge University Press 2011.

the landscape so that now the assessment of clinical skills is undertaken within local residency programmes in the context of national parameters.

The seismic shift in the venue of assessment has been accompanied by changes in the assessment procedures, issues of reliability and validity, questions about standards, and has resulted in greater attention to clinical skills training and assessment. It has also resulted in changes in the relationships between the major institutions involved in residency education – the ABPN, the American Council of Graduate Medical Education (ACGME), and the American Association of Directors of Psychiatric Residency Training (AADPRT).

The status quo

In psychiatry residency training in America, the ABPN (http://www.abpn.com/) is responsible for the certification of individual psychiatry residents, and influences residency training programmes only insofar as it defines specific aspects of the training experience that residents must have completed, in order to be eligible to sit for the board certification examination; for example, six months of inpatient rotations or 12 months of continuous outpatient care. But it is the Accreditation Council for Graduate Medical Education (ACGME, 2007), and its constituent specialty committees, that oversee the accreditation of residency programmes. Each specialty, psychiatry included, has a Residency Review Committee (RRC), which promulgates the Essential Requirements for residency programmes for that specialty based on a five-year cycle of review and revision. These detailed requirements, which comprise approximately 20–30 pages, describe all of the facets of the residency training, including rotation requirements, types of patient, programme resources, programme administration and necessary aspects of the departmental context. In recent years, these requirements have begun to reflect the attainment of educational competencies, and are no longer merely a compilation of required clinical educational experiences.

It falls upon the residency programme, and the programme director, to satisfy these twin masters – the ABPN and the ACGME with its Residency Review Committee – making sure that the programme conforms to the Essential Requirements and that graduating residents are eligible to sit for and perform successfully in the ABPN examination. This dual reporting structure is initially confusing to those not familiar with it but in fact there is relatively little confusion or conflict, as the functions of each of the overarching bodies are very clear and distinct. There is widespread consensus that adherence to the requirements of both organizations results in an optimal training experience. Furthermore, there is an appreciation of the redundancy involved, as programme directors regard preparation of their graduates for the ABPN examination to be a desirable goal, and most are pleased that the administration of the examination is separate from the training experience.

Programme directors generally appreciate the additional level of scrutiny their residents receive from ABPN examinations, freeing them from worry about either overly optimistic appraisals of their own residents, or from having to deliver bad news with serious career implications to trainees with whom they are closely connected. Although it is widely considered to have some problems and flaws, programme directors have viewed the ABPN examination as more objective than their own various in-residency assessments.

Until 2008, the board certification process involved two steps, both of which took place following residency training. Most residency graduates took the Part I written (computer-based in recent years) examination in the year or two following completion of their residency. This examination stresses medical knowledge and includes some clinical material. Successful completion of Part I allowed the psychiatrist to take Part II of the ABPN certification exam, which included both a live patient interview and an observed video interview. The live interview lasted 30 minutes and was followed by a 30-minute oral examination. The use of a semi-structured evaluation form led to a final grade. Next, observation of a video interview followed by oral examination provided some increased inter-rater reliability. There was a clear algorithm for determining the final pass or fail on the Part II examination based on the candidate's performance on these two components of the exam, with a small margin of judgement allowed to senior examiners if there was a marked discrepancy between the performance on the oral and video portions of the examination. As the shift to in-residency assessment has taken place, there has been a sequential phase-out of Part II of the examination and a modification of Part I.

There have been a variety of attempts to define and standardize the criteria for passing Part II of the ABPN certification process (McDermott et al., 1991; 1993). Teams observed the video interviews in advance, established benchmarks for performance and facilitated examiner consensus. There was extended discussion about the criteria for assessing the live patient interview, and examiners were trained in the types of questions and expected responses on the oral examination portions. Originally, two faculty members participated in each examination, and a senior examiner circulated among the rooms to help settle differences in grading. More recently, there was a switch to only one examiner, a change from qualitative grades to numerical ones, and the use of clinical vignettes instead of video interviews.

The two-part ABPN certification process was held in high esteem and it was a mark of honour to be invited to be an examiner for Part II. Examiners were selected by team leaders, who are national leaders in psychiatry, and typically participated in a team over a number of years and became quite affiliated with their group and with the ABPN examination enterprise.

Examiner interview techniques, perceptions of the standard for passing the exam, and indeed the whole ethos of the live patient and video interview became important aspects of the culture of psychiatric practice, psychiatric education, and indeed a part of professional identity formation for psychiatrists in America. For example, faculty members often reminded residents while on rotations about the appropriate way to handle clinical dilemmas, commenting on proper technique when it's time to 'take the Boards'.

Stimulus for change

This stable state of affairs changed after deliberations within the ABPN for the better part of a decade. Long-standing concerns about improving the reliability of the live patient interview, and to a lesser extent the video interview, resulted in the need for an examination format with greater inter-rater reliability. The cost of bringing together many examiners several times a year has risen dramatically, resulting in a substantial increase in the cost of the board certification examinations for recent graduates. There was increased interest in using new technology for delivering decision-tree-type examinations. Finally, there was a desire to provide an opportunity for remediation for those who have difficulty developing the competencies required for certification.

Board certification has become an increasingly important professional credential over the last 20 years. In earlier days, a minority of psychiatrists were certified, and certification was regarded as a distinction. More recently, the pressure for more effective and lower-cost care has led to greater systematization of mental health services, and Board certification is required by many mental health provider groups. Certification has gone from adding lustre to a professional's reputation to becoming an entry ticket for the job market.

A new model for clinical skills assessment

In 2008, the ABPN decided to phase out the live patient interview portion of the examination and require that psychiatry residency training programmes provide verification of clinical skills, which would allow graduates to sit for the Board examinations. Subsequently, they decided to eliminate the video interview, and collapse Parts I and II into a single comprehensive computer-administered examination, which would include assessment of medical knowledge and clinical application using interactive algorithms guiding questions about clinical vignettes.

The ABPN gave context for their decisions by calling attention to the rising expense and cumbersome logistics of the old-style exam, concerns about reliability, and the observation that in-residency clinical skills assessment would probably prove to be more effective and robust. The Board regarded in-residency assessment to be more consistent with competency-based training, an ACGME priority. The ABPN plans to maintain its traditional focus on certification in this new slimmed-down format, and increase its attention to the programme of re-certification, which requires that all ABPN-certified psychiatrists submit to practice-improvement activities and re-examination, every 10 years (Faulkner, 2008).

In response to the ABPN's new procedures, the Psychiatry Residency Review Committee of the ACGME made revisions in its Essential Requirements to accommodate these changes, including an intensified requirement for in-residency clinical skills assessment.

The ABPN's requirements for clinical skills assessment in residency were provided in a brief document that established the major parameters of the examination, but left many issues open (http://www.abpn.com/). This was done with the expectation that the programme directors would collaborate in developing effective models for assessment. The new assessment was referred to as 'clinical skills verification' (CSV).

These changes must also be understood in the context of the increased focus on competency-based medical training in America. Beginning in 2000, David Leach, MD, the CEO of the ACGME, laid out six essential competencies for graduate medical education: patient care, medical knowledge, practice-based learning, interpersonal and communication skills, professionalism, and systems-based practice (ACGME Outcome Project, http://www.acgme.org). Commitment to these competencies and their multifaceted and objective assessment has been the backbone of the ACGME's educational initiative since then. This has resulted in a substantial change in the focus of medical educators, with much greater attention to defining competencies and developing assessment tools for measuring trainees' competence. In a reference to the parallels between this process and the landmark national educational legislation of the Bush administration, entitled 'No Child Left Behind', the ACGME competency movement has been humorously referred to as 'No Resident Left Behind.'

The Residency Review Committee has been vigorously promoting competency-based training and including this in various ways in revisions of the Essential Requirements. With this background, the Residency Review Committee joined with the ABPN in highlighting clinical skills as a critical competency and mandated that residency programmes both teach competency and measure it in an effective and up-to-date manner.

Response from psychiatry residency training directors

Needless to say, these changes provoked controversy in residency training circles by establishing a new assessment mandate and setting aside a decades-old system of training, assessment and assignment of responsibility for each component of these activities.

The American Association of Directors of Psychiatry Residency Training (AADPRT), which represents 194 institutions, has in its membership 188 directors of adult psychiatry programmes, 110 directors of child and adolescent psychiatry training programmes, associate programme directors and quite a number of other sub-specialty training directors, became actively involved in this issue (http://www.aadprt.org/). Training directors questioned the reduced role of the ABPN, unsure of the implications of their stepping away from their traditional role of direct responsibility and accountability for the assessment of clinical skills. Programme directors were also concerned about the new and cumbersome assessments mandated for their programmes. They mourned the loss of the check-and-balance system, which required residents to satisfy both programme requirements and the ABPN live patient examination independently. Finally, they were concerned and confused by the lack of specificity in the ABPN requirement about the format of in-residency assessment of clinical skills.

The AADPRT appointed a Clinical Skills Task Force to study the issues and make recommendations about the appropriate interpretation and implementation of the new clinical skills verification mandate. There was a lively interchange between this task force and representatives from the ABPN and Residency Review Committee. Rather quickly the groups began to work effectively, with the Clinical Skills Task Force pushing for clarification about specifics, and the ABPN spelling out the minimum expected requirements for the clinical skills verification process. Indeed, the ABPN supported the task force in its task of framing recommendations for residency programmes about implementation of the new policy.

The ABPN CSV (clinical skills verification) requires that residents demonstrate competency in three areas: developing a doctor–patient relationship, clinical interviewing and case presentation. Each trainee must pass a minimum of three clinical assessments and meet the standard for competency in each of these areas in each assessment. The patients interviewed must be unfamiliar to the trainee, and the interview must be observed by faculty members who are ABPN-certified. The clinical interview is at least 30 minutes long, and is followed by a case presentation.

The ABPN defined the minimal level of competence required from the CSV as that of a practising psychiatrist in the community. The task force quickly recognized that the clinical skills assessments would need to take place early in the residency programme to allow for identification of trainees with skill deficits and the development of remediation programmes. The task force continues to struggle with the problem of squaring a competency definition that was based on psychiatrists in community practice with the competency level of trainees relatively early in training.

The ABPN allowed for significant flexibility in the assessment format. Assessments could take place in naturalistic settings, such as inpatient units, consultation liaison services, emergency rooms and outpatient clinics, or via ABPN 'board-style' interviews set up expressly for examination purposes.

The task force also struggled with the question of setting an appropriate pass rate for the clinical skills assessment process. It was clear that some trainees would not be able to demonstrate competence; in the current system, those same trainees might complete the programme and graduate. Other questions included how to define and implement remediation programmes, the design of grading forms for the assessment (which require ABPN approval), and practical problems in providing clinical skills verification for residents who go on to sub-specialty training. This last issue is especially thorny for child psychiatry, where residents have the option of 'fast tracking', meaning transferring to child and adolescent psychiatry training programmes after the third year of adult residency instead of going on to complete a fourth year. Finally, the task force took up the implication of CSV on the training of clinical skills.

New opportunities

The new clinical skills verification process and the change in roles of the ABPN, Residency Review Committee and psychiatry training programmes present several excellent opportunities for improving psychiatric education and assessment. When accrediting bodies require the re-conceptualization of an area of programme activity, this causes a flurry of activity and creative thought, and more resources are devoted to that area. We have already seen that the field has shone a spotlight on clinical skills training and assessment in the time since the ABPN foreshadowed their impending decision to implement clinical skills verification. These skills are widely regarded as the basic building blocks of good clinical care and there is no doubt that increased attention will improve our training. There is strong hope that the more formalized assessment procedures will help to identify residents with weaknesses in this area.

Ideally, the requirement for clinical skills verification will increase the degree of detailed observation of trainees' clinical interviewing and increase the amount of faculty time and attention to trainees' performance in this area. Identifying those residents who have difficulties will provide an opportunity for them to receive an individually tailored remediation programme, and hopefully a majority of these residents will successfully complete remediation and be able to improve their clinical skills to meet the requirement. Anecdotally, the increased attention to the assessments seems to result in more focus and discussion of the skills themselves, and indeed this may be an example of where 'teaching to the test' is desirable and beneficial.

The clinical skills verification process may turn out to be a leading example of how focusing on competencies and measuring them effectively changes education and changes outcome. In 2001, the Residency Review Committee mandated that residency programmes require competency in specific types of psychotherapy. This was required at a time when there was concern about psychotherapy training in residency programmes eroding and deteriorating. By defining those competencies and mandating their achievement, the committee achieved a significant success in reviving psychotherapy training, changing the field. We hope that the clinical skills verification will provoke a similar flowering of interest and attention, and thus allow for improvement of clinical training itself.

In-residency examination also offers the possibility of a better assessment process. The reliability and cost problems of the traditional ABPN Part II examination were discussed earlier. In addition to those issues, this 'high-stake' format results in increase in examinee anxiety and variance in outcome because of patient variability. Because the ABPN made clinical skills verification a requirement without specifying all of the particulars of the examination, there is an opportunity to make the procedure more effective. Specifically, there is an opportunity to assess clinical skills in a more naturalistic setting and examine them more frequently. The literature on performance-based assessments suggests that frequent briefer examinations are more reliable than less frequent, more extensive examinations, and clinical skills verification will allow us to take advantage of this observation (see Chapter 1). Finally, because the assessments are made in the context of an educational setting, they can be formative and not simply summative. If the assessments are made in a naturalistic rather than traditional 'board-style' setting, in the context of a clinical rotation, then they are more likely to be offered by teaching faculty and there may be more time for and a greater likelihood of constructive discussion and feedback.

Challenges

The new procedure for clinical skills verification will challenge programme directors to maintain their appropriate objectivity and be accountable for their trainees' clinical skills. Some programme directors have expressed concern about a 'conflict of interest', meaning that they will want their trainees to pass the examination and they may have a potential bias in the examination. However, the assessment of other aspects of resident performance has never been balanced by an external examination, such as the old Part II of the ABPN exam, and these assessments have not been regarded as tainted by conflicts of interest. Thus, there is much hope that 'conflict of interest' will not be a problem in the area of clinical skills assessment.

In general, competency-based education has been organized around developing specific competencies for trainees at each stage of training rather than monolithic competencies that cut across developmental phases. Yet, the clinical skills verification process reflects a single standard that does not depend on a trainee's level of training. Instead, it is pegged to the minimum competency of practising psychiatrists in the community. This is an unclear standard and individual faculty members and training programmes are uncertain how to apply it. Indeed, residency training directors as a group have been tasked by the ABPN with developing the standard. Some are concerned that the ABPN with its considerable resources, centralized authority, and time to work on this issue, was not able to achieve a significant consensus, i.e., enough inter-rater reliability. So how will it be possible for programmes and their faculty – more loosely organized and decentralized than the ABPN – to be able to do so?

There is very little known about how to design an effective remediation programme and very little data on measuring the impact of remediation. Thus, we are setting up a system that has as a virtue the early identification of those with a problem, yet we are unclear about the potential effectiveness of the response to that problem.

The passing rate for the CSV is yet another challenge. How many residents will not, and should not, pass the clinical skills assessment? What should happen to those residents? Some regard it as an advantage of the new procedure that those residents who are not able to obtain clinical skills credentials from the residency programme, despite remediation, should not go on to become practising psychiatrists. Yet, it is not clear what the workforce implications are of a procedure that weeds out more residents, nor the implications for the level of competence among psychiatrists in the field.

Because clinical skills verification must be completed while there is still time for remediation in the residency, and because a proportion of residents fast track into child psychiatry after their third year, the AADPRT Clinical Skills Task Force recommended that the assessments take place in the first and second postgraduate years. Thus, we are in the somewhat complicated position of teaching and then assessing a skill in early residency using a standard that we expect to be present among residency graduates. There is some worry that this will result in setting a bar that is too low. Those who take this position point out that clinical skills, i.e., the doctor–patient relationship, clinical interviewing and history presentation, are surely improved and honed during the third and fourth year of residency. They suggest that perhaps it is not reasonable to expect all residents to achieve an appropriate level of competency in two years when full training for this competency takes three or four years. Therefore, the CSV process may result in a 'watering down' of the competency standard. Those who disagree with this position point out that the clinical skills specified in the CSV are indeed fairly basic and that competent residents should be able to master them by the end of their second year. There are many other more sophisticated skills that residents develop during the third and fourth years of residency that are very important components of being a competent practising psychiatrist, but these are not what is tested in the CSV process.

The new ABPN mandate for clinical skills verification was supported and promptly included by the Residency Review Committee in a modification of the Essential Requirements in a striking example of convergence between these two institutions. This convergence represents an opportunity because close alignment of the ABPN and RRC will allow departments and training programme directors to function optimally, but there are worries that there will be a growing 'mono-lith' regulating residency training and that this may offer fewer opportunities for creativity and innovation.

Finally, the ABPN's new guidelines were not specific about the parameters of the clinical skills verification. This caused some degree of confusion among training directors. It is clear that the intent of this mandate is to stimulate some diversity and creativity in the field that will allow us to observe and study various ways of assessing clinical skills. This diversity will hopefully lead to a better end result, but there is some concern that it causes each programme to have to invest substantial resources in setting up the new assessment process.

Looking forward

Because of the generally understood need to develop an optimal format for implementing clinical skills verification programmes, and to begin to study and assess it, a unique multi-organizational task force was convened by the ABPN. Representatives from the ABPN, the RRC, the AADPRT, the American Academy of

Child Psychiatry, the American College of Psychiatrists and the Association for Academic Psychiatry met to share ideas and resources. This group's goal was to further define standards and develop a training workshop that would disseminate ideas and suggest procedures to the field.

The efforts of this working group culminated in the presentation of a workshop on clinical skills assessment at the AADPRT meeting of March 2009 with several hundred people present. This was followed by a presentation by the American Psychiatric Association in May 2009. The history of the CSV programme, the parameters of examination and some of the critical dilemmas and issues related to the examination were presented. This was followed by observation of several demonstration clinical interviews with rating of the doctor–patient relationship, clinical interviewing skills and patient presentation using an audience response system. This allowed the group an opportunity to develop some very preliminary consensus on the competency standards in each of the three designated areas. All of these materials, including the videos and group ratings, were subsequently put on the organization's website in a downloadable format so that individual directors can use them to train their faculties. There are plans for statistical evaluation and publication of this data.

The ABPN retains an important monitoring function for clinical skills verification in residencies, but has stepped out of the process of examination development, faculty training and assessment. The ABPN Task Force on Clinical Skills Verification Rater Training and the AADPRT Clinical Skills Task Force continue their work in both developing resources for the examination and monitoring developments in the field. It is anticipated that there will be a survey to gather data on how programmes are conducting their assessments and what their experience has been.

Ultimately, the important questions regarding in-residency clinical skills assessment remain to be answered. How much will in-residency assessment improve clinical skills training? What kinds of testing formats will programmes use, and will there be an evolution towards more naturalistic assessment settings? To what degree will a consensus develop on the bar for competency for clinical skills? How effective will remediation be for residents who are found to be deficient? What will the pass rate be? How much inter-rater reliability will there be within and between programmes? Of course, the most important larger question is whether clinical skills verification will improve psychiatry residency training and the competence of psychiatrists in the future.

REFERENCES

ACGME Program Requirements for Graduate Medical Education in Psychiatry (2007). http://www.acgme.org/acWebsite/downloads/RRC_progReq/400_psychiatry_07012007_u04122008.pdf.

Faulkner, L. R. (2008). Update on the ABPN Maintenance of Certification Program and the ABPN's Certification Examinations. *ABPN Update*, **14**, 1–4.

McDermott, J. F., Jr, Tanguay, P. E., Scheiber, S. C. *et al.* (1991). Reliability of the Part II board certification examination in psychiatry: interexaminer consistency. *American Journal of Psychiatry*, **148**, 1672–1674.

McDermott, J. F., Jr, Tanguay, P. E., Scheiber, S. C. *et al.* (1993). Reliability of the Part II board certification examination in psychiatry: examination stability. *American Journal of Psychiatry*, **150**, 1077–1080.

8

Determining competence of psychiatric residents in the USA

Joan Anzia and John Manring

Editors' introduction

Following on from the previous chapter, where Richard Summers describes the national changes occurring in the United States Postgraduate Psychiatric Assessments, Joan Anzia and John Manring outline the manner in which local training programme directors have responded to these changes. There are examples of local and national collaboration amongst programme directors to produce innovative methods of assessing trainee performance and some of these are outlined in this chapter. There are accounts of the development of workplace-based assessment tools and processes by programme directors, who have harnessed their educational and professional expertise to create performance-based assessment programmes that are aimed at fulfilling both the developmental and decision-making needs of assessments in postgraduate training.

Introduction

As Richard Summers described in Chapter 7, medical education in the USA is extraordinarily complex and often fragmented because of the sheer number of stakeholders involved and the hierarchy of their different goals and values. In our academic culture, the process of medical education is divided into discrete segments of training, producing a patchwork progression rather than the ideal seamless voyage from undergraduate (college or university) education, through medical school, residency, fellowship, state licensure, attending psychiatrist status and finally Board certification. Darryl Kirch MD, President of the Association of American Medical Colleges, stated at the 2009 Meeting of the Association for Academic Psychiatry, 'We need to create a true continuum that is seamless.'

Workplace-Based Assessments in Psychiatric Training, ed. Dinesh Bhugra and Amit Malik.
Published by Cambridge University Press. © Cambridge University Press 2011.

Although there is collaboration between some of these schools, programmes and organizations (especially between the ACGME, the RRC and the ABPN) they frequently have differing visions and goals. Studies of graduate medical education programmes that are most successful in terms of innovation and learning outcomes indicate that one important component is a centralized educational structure that is 'tight and coherent' (Philibert *et al.*, 2010). The relative lack of coherence among stakeholder agencies in the USA may be a very real impediment to improvement. A psychiatry training director in the United States must understand and adhere to the regulations and expectations of all of these different bodies, and this has made the process of educational change at the programme level particularly challenging.

Our purpose in this chapter is to describe the process of recent changes in US psychiatric residency education from the viewpoint of the training director, with a special focus on evaluation and assessment. We will describe the range of tools and assessment settings that are currently used in US training programmes, training directors' struggles to meet new competency and assessment requirements of accrediting bodies, and some promising innovations in individual programmes.

Description of the stakeholders

A brief and basic overview of the network of certifying and accrediting bodies from the training director's viewpoint is necessary in order to understand the competing forces at play in this change process (Table 8.1).

While the mission of the American Association of Directors of Psychiatric Residency Training (AADPRT) is to 'promote excellence in the education and training of future psychiatrists' (AADPRT, 2010a), early in its development the organization came to serve the interests of training directors as well (AADPRT, 2010b). It is the central 'home base' where they seek information, guidance and support. This is an organization of several hundred training directors who meet together annually, compare notes via an organizational email mailing list and send representatives to other stakeholder organizations. Although the AADPRT does not serve in any accrediting or certifying roles, its members have input into decisions by the accrediting and certifying organizations (AADPRT, 2010b). The AADPRT meetings are an important venue in which training directors share observations, opinions, educational innovations and research.

Training prior to 2001

In Chapter 7, Richard Summers described the beginning of the ACGME 'Outcome Project' that began in 2001 with the introduction of the six 'competencies' for American graduate medical education. Assessment of competence in American psychiatry residency programmes prior to 2001 was primarily left to the

Table 8.1 An overview of US accrediting bodies

Organization	Acronym	Role
Accreditation Council for Graduate Medical Education	ACGME	Evaluates and accredits all graduate medical education programmes in the USA. Sets standards for medical education and introduced the concept and structure of 'competencies'
Psychiatry Residency Review Committee of the ACGME	RRC	Develops programme requirements for psychiatry residency programmes in the USA
American Association of Directors of Psychiatric Residency Training	AADPRT	Voluntary organization of American psychiatry programme directors
American Board of Psychiatry and Neurology	ABPN	Division of the American Board of Medical Specialties, which evaluates graduates of training programmes for individual 'Board certification' in psychiatry and neurology
Federation of State Medical Boards	FSMB	Organization of all the licensing bodies of individual American states that distribute medical licences

training director of each individual programme. Written general evaluations of the resident's progress in a clinical rotation were submitted to the training director by faculty supervisors at the end of each rotation. There was no standard format for feedback or evaluation forms. Some programmes had forms that were quite lengthy and elaborate; other forms were brief and very concrete. Some programmes emphasized in-depth learning in psychodynamic psychotherapy in their forms, for example, and others emphasized diagnostic skills and somatic therapies. Often, the evaluation forms reflected the orientation or interests of the particular department or training director. In a larger context, the different emphases in varying programmes reflected a lack of consensus in American academic psychiatry about what defined a psychiatrist's essential knowledge and skills. This lack of definition of 'minimal competency' in psychiatry was so pronounced that for many years new ABPN Board Examiners were never given explicit definitions of what constituted a 'passing performance'. Two other evaluations were common to most programmes but not required. These were the Psychiatry Resident-In-Training Examination (PRITE), a multiple-choice-question knowledge examination given annually in most programmes (created by yet another professional organization, the American College of Psychiatrists), and 'mock board' clinical skill exams, given at least once by the majority of programmes in the final year of training, but two or three times on an annual basis in many programmes. This latter examination involved a live patient interview followed by a presentation of the residents' find-ings to the examiners and an oral examination of diagnosis, formulation and treatment.

Nor was there any required training in feedback and evaluation for faculty super-visors. The RRC had long required that each programme have a Residency Train-ing Committee, composed of the training and fellowship directors and key faculty members, which was to meet regularly to monitor resident progress, evaluate the programme and resolve programmatic issues that arose. In many programmes this committee provided a 'checks-and-balances' function in the evaluation of res-idents, a kind of primitive form of calibration through mutual discussion of the resident's performance.

Until 2007 there was no requirement for observation and evaluation of specific clinical skills except for the 'mock board' exam, which was required twice during the training years. Since the 'mock board' examination was administered in a format similar to that of the Part II ABPN 'live-patient' exams, it was generally used more as a 'formative' examination to prepare the resident for the ABPN summative examination. The faculty examiners for the 'mock board' rated the resident according to a form created by the individual residency programme, and often gave feedback to the resident directly after the presentation. The 'mock board' examination was not summative, nor was it used to make final decisions about promotion or graduation of residents. If a resident failed a 'mock board' exam, there was no generally prescribed remediation that a programme was required to implement. Faculty members generally received no training in evaluating residents, and often they were familiar with the residents from clinical rotations. The 'mock board' proved modestly reliable in predicting a pass on the ABPN oral examination ($p = 0.03$) but not at predicting failure in passing the ABPN examination in a study of 10 years of experience at one medium-sized programme (J. Manring, J. Salvagno, L. Profenno, unpublished data).

The beginning of change

In 2001, when the first phase of the new ACGME Outcome Project was introduced to psychiatry training directors, with its six core competencies (patient care, med-ical knowledge, professionalism, systems-based practice, practice-based learning and improvement, interpersonal and communication skills (ACGME, 2005)), the requirements for learning experiences in all competencies, the improvement of evaluation forms, and the aggregate data on resident improvement, it was greeted with a mixture of excitement, confusion, great concern, and in some cases, anger. Many directors were very worried that they would not have the time or resources to meet all the requirements within the ACGME timeline. Initially, not many examples of curricula or evaluation tools were available as models. Training direc-tors felt that however laudable the ACGME's mission of change, the burden of implementation had fallen squarely on their shoulders.

In fairly short order, however, groups of psychiatric educators began to publish and post ideas for developing different clinical experiences, evaluation forms, and innovative assessment tools. The ACGME created a 'toolbox' of suggested methods and forms (ACGME, 2000), and the AADPRT website made available a growing number of portable curricula and assessment forms, all of which could be downloaded by members of the AADPRT for general use. Training directors also frequently shared information, ideas and moral support via the AADPRT listserve messageboard; this medium has played a central role during the process of change.

By 2006, most, if not all, American training programmes had written curricular goals and objectives for each of the competency domains, and evaluation forms for clinical rotations were written in the language and format of the six 'competencies'. Residency directors were evaluating their educational programmes on an annual basis, and developing programme improvement plans based on resident performance. By 2009, most programmes had adopted multiple assessments during training (at least two per competency as mandated by the new requirements). In addition to the summative rotation evaluations, most programmes now use a variety of assessments which include various mixes of:

- Semi-annual '360-degree' evaluations of trainees' professionalism and communication/interpersonal skills (from nursing, social work, and psychology staff as well as patients);
- Multiple assessments of knowledge (for example, a multiple-choice examination about cognitive-behavioural therapy or psychodynamic psychiatry, such as the Columbia Psychodynamic Psychotherapy Exam, in addition to the PRITE exam);
- Chart-stimulated recall assessments that evaluate clinical decision-making;
- Semi-annual resident self-assessments of learning goals and objectives.

To our knowledge, no-one has yet published a comprehensive survey of the assessments currently being used by US psychiatry training programmes. Anecdotal information based on contributions to the AADPRT listserve messageboard suggests that the variation extant prior to 2001 has continued to some degree in both quantity and quality of assessment processes, evaluation tools and faculty training in our programmes. In some programmes the 'letter of the law' of the ACGME has been implemented in terms of competency language in curricula and forms, but the occurrence of genuine educational change is questionable. The overwhelming emphasis on development of the appropriate language and format in these initial stages led Joel Yager, one of the leading American psychiatric educators, to warn the 2006 national meeting of the Association for Academic Psychiatry of the dangers of losing sight of the larger mission of quality education through immersion in the details of the 'competency-industrial complex'.

The second phase of change: the clinical skills verification exams

As the first phase of the ACGME Outcome Project progressed, training directors were faced with a second major change. For many decades, the ABPN had provided a pair of summative exams, a written multiple-choice examination (Part I) the successful completion of which qualified one to proceed to the oral examination of a live patient interview (Part II), the successful completion of which led to 'Board certification' of the individual psychiatrist. In 2007, the ABPN announced that it would be phasing out its Part II oral examination. In its place, residency programmes would be required to conduct a series of in-training clinical skills examinations so that residents could be 'credentialed' to take the Board certification written examination. There would no longer be any independent summative evaluation of clinical skills as part of ABPN exams, only a computerized multiple-choice examination.

Training directors initially responded to this decision with varying degrees of consternation, frustration and some anger. Firstly, despite the generally acknowledged flaws of the Part II exam, it provided some assurance that residency graduates would have a summative assessment of the most important skills of the psychiatrist: conducting a diagnostic interview while developing rapport with a patient, recognizing diagnostic phenomena and presenting the case with a list of differential diagnoses and treatment plans. Secondly, the Part II examination was conducted by someone with no conflict of interest in the outcome. And finally, training directors were now expected to shoulder the task of providing for summative assessment of clinical skills that had once been the purview of the APBN.

The details for the new regimen were presented as follows: all residents who began their first postgraduate year after July 2007 must satisfactorily pass three clinical skills verification examinations (Appendix 8.1 shows a sample CSV form) in the early years of training to be eligible for Board certification. The examinations are to consist of an actual live patient interview at least 30 minutes in length, followed by an oral case presentation. The patient must be unknown to the resident, and the faculty examiner must be Board certified. The three passing examinations must have been conducted with at least two different faculty examiners. The standard for passing the examination is a performance equal to that expected from a competent psychiatrist practising in the community. The examination can be held in a variety of settings: at a clinical site as part of a rotation, in the old 'mock board' format, or in a workshop setting, and the resident may take the examination any number of times. The residency programmes may use forms provided by the ABPN and AADPRT, or they may submit their own form for approval to the ABPN. The form must include evaluation of the physician–patient relationship, conduct of interview and case presentation. As part of this process, the ABPN partnered with the ACGME's Psychiatry RRC to ensure that all residency programmes are required to provide the clinical skills verification examinations as described.

What was the 'Part II exam'? As already described in Chapter 7, the examination that was commonly called the 'Oral Boards' in American psychiatry consisted of a high-stakes, high-anxiety professional hurdle: a 30-minute live interview of a patient, followed by a 30-minute case presentation of findings and discussion of diagnosis, formulation and treatment plan conducted for most examinees in an unfamiliar location, if not an unfamiliar city. The interview was observed by two experienced Board examiners unfamiliar with either the examinee or the patient. The second part of that oral examination used to consist of a videotape clip of a patient interview unfamiliar to either the examiner or candidate, after which the candidate presented the case and discussed diagnosis and treatment with the examiners. The pass rate for the examination hovered between 60% and 70%. Board certification is not currently required for the practice of psychiatry in most settings in the USA, but is seen as a mark of excellence and often ensures a higher salary in academic departments as well as most other organizations. Residency training programmes with high 'board pass rates' often published these results as an indication of their programme excellence.

Problems with the Part II ABPN examination included flaws in inter-rater reliability, a low level of standardization, few data points, high expense, unfamiliar surroundings and immense logistical complexity. However, the examination did have a significant element of face validity, as it tested crucial clinical skills. In 2004, the ABPN attempted to increase the number of data points and improve standardization by substituting four 12-minute vignette stations for the single video part of the examination. Three of the vignettes were written cases with four questions; one was a video clip of an actual patient with four questions. The initial vignettes were quite basic, leaving many examiners worried about the meaningfulness of the examination in assessing graduate psychiatrists. The examiner read a short case vignette about a single patient and the examinee tasks were restricted to presenting the mental status examination or discussing the diagnosis, treatment options or potential challenges in the therapeutic relationship.

Faculty evaluator training initiative

In addition, the ABPN gathered a group of representatives from most of the stakeholder organizations to discuss training for faculty evaluators of the examinations. This workgroup, the ABPN Task Force on Clinical Skills Verification Rater Training, met several times throughout 2007 and 2008 to review literature on evaluator training, practice frame-of-reference and performance dimension training, and plan live and online training modules for faculty. An initial three-hour live training session was conducted in a large auditorium at the AADPRT annual meeting in Tucson, Arizona in March of 2009, where residency training directors and other psychiatric educators viewed sample videotapes of resident interviews and case presentations, and engaged in frame-of-reference and performance dimension training through the use of audience response system technology and live discussion between videotapes. This workshop was repeated at the annual meeting of the American Psychiatric Association in May 2009 and the annual meeting of the Association for Academic Psychiatry in October 2009. Data from these training sessions are currently being aggregated, but preliminary reports indicate that there was generally good consensus on judgement of competency in resident interviews (personal communication, Michael Jibson, MD and Karen Broquet, MD, Chairpersons, ABPN Task Force on Clinical Skills Verification Rater Training).

The PowerPoint presentations, the video clips and the rating forms are posted on the AADPRT website for use by training directors. Although neither the ABPN nor the Psychiatry RRC currently require faculty training for the clinical skills verification examinations, they both encourage this training at national meetings, online, and in individual departments of psychiatry.

By 2013, the summative evaluation of clinical skills of psychiatry trainees in the United States will occur solely within the individual residency training programmes; there will be no national summative evaluation. In Chapter 7, Dr Summers has listed many of the unanswered questions about the details of the new process. What format will most programmes use to perform the exams? What if a resident is unable to pass the three CSV examinations even after several attempts? What kinds of remediation will be available for such trainees? How will profession-wide standards be safeguarded when individual training directors are 'signing off' on trainees' clinical competence, especially as training directors are at times under pressure to graduate residents on time (without extending stipends for residents who need remediation)? Is conflict-of-interest or familiarity a problem when faculty members who train residents also serve as evaluators for exams? An unpublished study, presented by John Manring at the national meeting of the APA in 2008, comparing mock board examination outcomes with ABPN outcomes over the past 10 years at one medium-sized programme found that eight of nine failing performances on mock boards were identified by examiners who were visiting faculty from another programme, a result which did not reach statistical significance but was alarming nonetheless. All of these questions are ripe for inquiry and investigation in the near future.

The AADPRT and other stakeholder organizations are encouraging programmes to administer the clinical skills verification examinations early and often in training in order to encourage growing familiarity with the examination (in trainees and faculty), to accustom trainees to the experience of 'not passing', and to increase the opportunity for formative feedback and skill improvement. Based on an early informal AADPRT listserve messageboard inquiry in the autumn of 2009, programme directors who responded are requiring that residents take the CSV examinations from twice a month to once every three months, and are choosing to have trainees take the examinations in the daily course of their clinical rotations, with their clinical site faculty members as evaluators. Some programmes are continuing to hold annually scheduled examination days, in the old 'mock board' format.

As yet there has been no formal survey of trainees' responses to the new exams, but anecdotal input from several training directors suggests that psychiatry residents in the USA, who are used to many previous high-stake pass–fail exams, need some time to adjust to a culture of constructive feedback and improvement when they do not 'pass' the CSV examination at their first attempts. For our trainees, the experience of taking a summative examination that they will most probably initially fail marks an encounter with a new culture in their medical education. For American faculty, the experience of 'failing' so many beginning trainees in an examination is also a new experience, and they, too, require support in adopting their new roles.

Beginnings of innovation in assessment: suggestions for the future

We will review a few of the innovative projects in assessment in US residency programmes. Many American medical schools have built, or are planning to build, simulation centres for all levels of medical education. Although medical specialties with many procedures – such as surgery and anaesthesia – have embraced technology in education and have long-established routine simulation training and assessment, American psychiatric education has primarily used standardized patients (SPs) for summative examinations in medical school, not residency training. In our view, US training directors must also learn to utilize simulation and other educational technologies for learning and assessment. The validity and reliability of standardized patient simulations in medical education has been well-established over the past 30 years (Satish *et al.*, 2009).

Strategic management simulation (SMS)

A particularly sophisticated use of simulation technology has been successfully applied for decades to evaluate and train leaders in industry and the military in decision-making under circumstances characterized by volatility, uncertainty, complexity, ambiguity and delayed feedback (VUCAD). More recently, this technology is being applied in medical training. The SMS system records and quantifies several subtle components of functioning that have been hard to measure, such as communication, teamwork, utilization of knowledge, integration, use of planning and strategy and follow-up of results that accumulate with decisions. Participants make decisions during the simulation task period, for example, the time following the hand-off of information when beginning an overnight call. The absence of requirements to engage in specific actions or to make decisions at specific points in time, the absence of stated demands to respond to specific information, the freedom to develop initiative, and the freedom for strategy development and decision implementation allow participants to utilize their own preferred or typical actions, using their preferred planning and strategic styles. The real-world atmosphere of the task and setting, involving several potentially interactive components of task demands as well as many interactive options to engage in various aspects of behaviour allows for a realistic assessment of competence.

Measurement using the simulation technique provides both numeric and graphic information on competence across a range of responses to task demands. Assessed performance attributes on 25 validated performance indicators vary from 'simpler' measures of competency in categories such as 'activity' and 'timeliness of response', through categories such as 'information orientation', 'information utilization' and 'emergency management' to increasingly complex measures in such areas of functioning as 'initiative', 'breadth of approach to challenges', 'planning', 'strategy' and so forth.

The unique aspect of this measurement technology is its ability to define broad parameters of decision-making in specific terms. For example, overall activity level is measured not just in terms of all the activity evident in the simulation but also measured in terms of its specific focus to a particular task and its application to overall goals (Satish et al., 2009).

Twenty-five psychiatry residents at SUNY Upstate Medical University participated in an SMS. Two standardized tests, the Psychiatry Resident-In-Training Examination (PRITE) and the Columbia Psychodynamic Psychotherapy Skills Test (CPPST), as well as faculty evaluations, were used to compare performance. The faculty evaluation scale included a series of questions that help rate the resident's competence in, for example, 'actual' patient management, communication skills, and emergency management. The two standardized tests used, the PRITE and the CPPST, were well-correlated with each other; however, these tests did not predict actual resident performance as observed by faculty. Several simulation measures correlated higher with faculty ratings than PRITE and Columbia Psychotherapy scores. The SMS scores proved a better reflection of resident performance than standard tests (Satish et al., 2009).

It is significant that simulation data were obtained during a two-hour simulation. In contrast, faculty ratings did not stabilize until at least two years after the residents had joined the department. Even then, it was not always clear to faculty what aspect of functioning impaired performance, yet the simulation measures identified specific performance deficits. In contrast to assessment with the two standardized tests, simulation performance values are highly stable over time and can be obtained at any time (e.g., immediately after entry into a residency programme) and reflect different specific components of resident competence. Information obtained about the individual resident's strengths and weaknesses in decision-making and problem-solving can be used for focused feedback and training or remediation to enhance subsequent performance. The SMS thereby represents an especially powerful tool for both formative and summative evaluation of residents, a tool that can guide a resident's further training.

Simulation of psychiatric emergencies

Art Walaszek, MD, the psychiatry training director at the University of Wisconsin School of Medicine, has designed a pilot simulation curriculum on managing behavioural emergencies for first- and second-year residents. The curriculum consists of a series of short vignettes in which a resident engages a 'patient' in an emergency room or inpatient setting. The goal of the curriculum is to provide formative feedback on a resident's evaluation of an emergent clinical situation, choice of strategies and implementation of skills. The clinical situations include acute suicidality, acute psychosis or mania, and substance intoxication and withdrawal. Residents must pass six evaluations (two each) to graduate from needing direct supervision of all patient interactions. These skills are phase-appropriate learning targets in the first years of training and are fairly easily measured. (The assessment forms are given in Appendices 8.2 to 8.4).

Developing standards and assessments in professionalism in psychiatry

West *et al.* (2007) described educational goals for professionalism and discussed the challenges with assessment of professionalism given current commonly utilized tools in residency education. They point out that competencies for professionalism in psychiatry that are measurable and attainable have been developed; the next step is the creation of valid and feasible assessment tools. Simulated clinical vignettes could assess whether a trainee 'knows how' to perform professionally, while different tools would be necessary to measure what he or she 'does' in the daily practice of psychiatry.

In summary, there are many innovative pilot curricula and some new assessment tools in American psychiatric education, but we have yet to provide solid, consistent links between improvements in residency education and quality patient care. Projects for the future include:

1. A comprehensive survey of the assessment methods and outcome data of American psychiatry residency programmes,
2. A comprehensive survey of the formats, frequency and outcomes of the new clinical skills verification examinations,
3. A study examining the impact of conflicts of interest in the clinical skills verification examinations,
4. Methods of measuring the outcome of innovative curricula in such areas as residents-as-teachers, residents as culturally competent, residents as competent practitioners of evidence-based psychiatry, residents as competent in ethical dilemmas unique to psychiatry (such as capacity decisions), and competency in procedures such as ECT and perhaps rTMS.

APPENDIX 8.1 AADPRT CLINICAL SKILLS VERIFICATION EXAMINATION FORM

AADPRT Clinical Skills Verification Examination Form CSV.3

Resident _____   PGY _____

Examiner _____   Date _____

Complexity of Patient _____   Difficulty of Interview _____

Directions: Complete the subscore worksheet on pages 2-5 using the anchors shown. An **overall** score of 5 or more is required for an acceptable performance on the 3 major items below. Please note that these scores are for overall performance in each area; the resident is not required to pass each sub-item. Anchors for patient complexity and interview difficulty are on page 6.

1. Physician Patient Relationship	Overall score _____	☐ Acceptable ☐ Unacceptable

2. Conduct of the Interview	Overall score _____	☐ Acceptable ☐ Unacceptable

3. Case Presentation	Overall score _____	☐ Acceptable ☐ Unacceptable

Comments:

_____   _____
Examiner Signature   Resident Signature

(Version CSV.3, revised 3/17/08)

AADPRT Clinical Skills Verification Worksheet

1. Physician Patient Relationship

☐ Acceptable: Overall score is ≥5

Overall Score _____

☐ Unacceptable: Overall score is ≤4

1-1. Develops rapport with patient

Excellent:	Courteous, professional demeanor	☐ 8
	Clear introduction to patient	
	Exhibits warmth and empathy	☐ 7
Good:	Generally respectful	☐ 6
	Adequate introduction	
	Adequate empathy	☐ 5
Fair:	Arrogant, disrespectful, or awkward demeanor	☐ 4
	Inadequate introduction	
	Lacks empathy	☐ 3
Poor:	Rude or inappropriate comments	☐ 2
	No introduction or misrepresentation of the situation	
	Obvious anger or frustration	☐ 1

1-2. Responds appropriately to patient

Excellent:	Responds empathically to verbal and nonverbal cues	☐ 8
	Adjusts interview to patient's level of understanding and cultural background	
	Adjusts interview to new information	☐ 7
Good:	Responds adequately to verbal and nonverbal cues	☐ 6
	Occasional use of technical jargon	
	Adjusts interview to most new information	☐ 5
Fair:	Shows minimal response to sensitive information	☐ 4
	Minimal awareness of patient's capacity to understand or cultural background	
	Inflexible interviewing style	☐ 3
	Misses important verbal and nonverbal cues	
Poor:	Responds with angry, abusive, or dismissive comments	☐ 2
	Frequently loses composure	
	Criticizes, demeans, or condemns patient	☐ 1

1-3. Follows cues presented by patient

Excellent:	Responds appropriately to verbal and nonverbal information	☐ 8
	Follows up on all pertinent information	
	Seeks clarification of ambiguous information	☐ 7
Good:	Misses no major verbal or nonverbal information	☐ 6
	Generally follows up on major issues presented by the patient	
		☐ 5
Fair:	Misses significant verbal and nonverbal information	☐ 4
	Fails to ask for clarification of ambiguous information	
		☐ 3
Poor:	Ignores or responds inappropriately to verbal or nonverbal cues	☐ 2
	Grossly misinterprets verbal or nonverbal information	
		☐ 1

2. Conduct of the Interview

Overall Score _____

☐ Acceptable: Overall score is ≥5

☐ Unacceptable: Overall score is ≤4

2-1. Obtains sufficient data for DSM Axes I-V differential diagnosis

Excellent:	Assists the patient in describing the full range of symptoms and history	☐ 8
	Explores all pertinent domains of information	
	Gathers adequate information for DSM checklists	☐ 7
Good:	Allows patient to describe major symptoms and history	☐ 6
	Explores the major domains of information	
	Focuses interview on DSM checklists	☐ 5
Fair:	Limits interview to DSM checklists	☐ 4
	Misses important domains of information	
	Shows little awareness or regard for DSM diagnoses	☐ 3
	Fails to consider alternative diagnoses	
Poor:	Fails to gather sufficient information for major diagnosis	☐ 2
	Misinterprets or misrepresents diagnostic information	
		☐ 1

2-2. Obtains psychiatric, medical, substance use, family, and social histories

Excellent:	Assists the patient in presenting each aspect of the history	☐ 8
	Gathers a wide range of biopsychosocial information	
	Maintains focus and logical progression of interview	☐ 7
	Appears comfortable with difficult or sensitive topics	
Good:	Allows the patient to present an adequate range of material	☐ 6
	Gathers adequate biopsychosocial information	
	Generally redirects the patient when necessary	☐ 5
	Somewhat uncomfortable with difficult or sensitive topics	
Fair:	Interrupts or interferes with the patient's story	☐ 4
	Misses important biopsychosocial information	
	Fails to redirect or focus a disorganized or hyperverbal patient	☐ 3
	Avoids difficult or sensitive topics	
Poor:	Ignores pertinent areas of the history	☐ 2
	Asks cursory, disorganized, or irrelevant questions	
	Loses control of the interview	☐ 1
	Responds inappropriately to difficult or sensitive topics	

2-3. Screens for suicidality, homicidality, high risk behavior, and trauma

Excellent:	Approaches topic frankly, but with sensitivity and empathy	☐ 8
	Asks questions appropriate to the context of the interview	
	Follows up with specific questions	☐ 7
	Assesses specific suicide risk factors, if relevant	
Good:	Approaches topic somewhat awkwardly	☐ 6
	Asks general screening questions	
	Follows up with 1-2 specific questions	☐ 5
Fair:	Approaches topic with abrupt, accusatory, or incredulous manner	☐ 4
	Asks only indirect or cursory questions	
	Obtains no detailed information	☐ 3
Poor:	Fails to address suicidal or homicidal ideation	☐ 2
	Disregards pertinent information in the history regarding patient's risk factors	
		☐ 1

2-4. Uses open- and close-ended questions

Excellent:	Uses frequent, well-structured open-ended questions Balances open and closed questions	□ 8 □ 7
Good:	Uses occasional open-ended questions	□ 6 □ 5
Fair:	Interview consists primarily of directive, closed-ended questions	□ 4 □ 3
Poor:	Interview consists entirely of narrowly focused, closed-ended questions	□ 2 □ 1

2-5. Performs an adequate mental status examination

Excellent:	All pertinent areas of the MSE were addressed Appropriate areas of the MSE were integrated into other parts of the interview	□ 8 □ 7
Good:	Most pertinent areas of the MSE were addressed Occasional areas of the MSE were integrated into other parts of the interview	□ 6 □ 5
Fair:	At least one essential element of the MSE was omitted	□ 4 □ 3
Poor:	Multiple elements of the MSE were omitted	□ 2 □ 1

3. Case Presentation

Overall Score _____

☐ Acceptable: Overall score is ≥5

☐ Unacceptable: Overall score is ≤4

3-1. Organized and accurate presentation of history

Excellent:	HPI accurately reflects the patient's story	☐ 8
	Presentation is logical, concise, and coherent	
	History integrates all important biopsychosocial factors	
	Presentation includes pertinent positive and negative findings	☐ 7
	Presentation leads to a clear understanding of the patient	
Good:	HPI generally reflects the patient's story	☐ 6
	Presentation can be followed	
	History includes adequate discussion of biopsychosocial factors	
	Presentation includes major pertinent negative findings	☐ 5
	Presentation leads to an adequate understanding of the patient	
Fair:	HPI ignores or inaccurately represents the patient's story	☐ 4
	Presentation is disorganized or chaotic	
	History misses important biopsychosocial factors	
	Presentation ignores some pertinent positive or negative findings	☐ 3
	Presentation leads to a poor understanding of the patient	
Poor:	HPI distorts or misinterprets the patient's story	☐ 2
	Presentation is incoherent or illogical	
	History shows no awareness of biopsychosocial issues	
	Presentation misinterprets or disregards pertinent positive or negative findings	☐ 1
	Presentation is grossly inaccurate	

3-2. Organized and accurate presentation of mental status findings

Excellent:	All areas of the MSE are presented	☐ 8
	Presentation is orderly, systematic, and easy to follow	
	Standard terminology and nomenclature are used	
	Findings are accurate and complete	
	Pertinent negative findings are included	☐ 7
	An appropriate and accurate assessment of dangerousness is included	
Good:	Most areas of the MSE are presented	☐ 6
	Presentation generally follows a standard outline	
	Clear and meaningful terms are used	
	All critical findings are included	
	Most important negative findings are included	☐ 5
	An adequate assessment of dangerous is included	
Fair:	Several pertinent areas of the MSE are omitted	☐ 4
	Presentation is disorganized and rambling	
	Ambiguous, inappropriate, or unclear terminology is used	
	Some critical findings are omitted or misrepresented	
	Important negative findings are omitted	☐ 3
	Assessment of dangerousness is inadequate or only partially accurate	
Poor:	Major areas of the MSE are omitted	☐ 2
	Presentation is incoherent and impossible to follow	
	Inaccurate, meaningless, or inappropriate terminology is used	
	Most critical findings are omitted or misrepresented	
	Negative findings are not included	☐ 1
	Assessment of dangerousness is omitted or is inaccurate	

Complexity of Patient

☐ Low: Patient presents one primary problem with clearly described symptoms

☐ Medium: Patient presents one problem with vaguely or inconsistently described symptoms
              or 2-3 problems with clear symptoms

☐ High: Patient presents multiple problems with vaguely or inconsistently described
              symptoms

Difficulty of Interview

☐ Low: Patient is cooperative, well organized, and cognitively intact

☐ Medium: Patient is abrupt, uncertain, or cognitively compromised

☐ High: Patient is hostile, disorganized, or cognitively impaired

APPENDIX 8.2 ASSESSMENT FORM FOR 'ACUTE SUICIDALITY'

University of Wisconsin Psychiatry Residency
Evaluation of Basic Emergency Psychiatry Skills (Accompanied Call)
ACUTE SUICIDALITY

Resident:_____   Date:_____
Attending:_____

Behavioural objectives: assessment	N/A	Not Done	Done: needs improvement	Done: meets expectations
Culturally sensitive and empathic	☐	☐	☐	☐
Establishes and maintains rapport	☐	☐	☐	☐
Focused and efficient interview	☐	☐	☐	☐
Depressive symptoms	☐	☐	☐	☐
Suicidal ideation, including plan, intent and means	☐	☐	☐	☐
Access to means of suicide	☐	☐	☐	☐
Any recent self-harm behaviour of any type	☐	☐	☐	☐
Psychiatric sx: anxiety, psychosis, substance use, homicidality	☐	☐	☐	☐
Recent psychosocial stressors and precipitants	☐	☐	☐	☐
Support systems and protective factors	☐	☐	☐	☐
Past psychiatric history, including review of medical records	☐	☐	☐	☐
Concurrent medical problems and medication use	☐	☐	☐	☐
If patient has harmed self: any medical complications	☐	☐	☐	☐
Relevant developmental history	☐	☐	☐	☐
MSE, including cognition	☐	☐	☐	☐
Collateral information to corroborate history	☐	☐	☐	☐
Prelim. biopsychosocial formulation and DSM-IV axial diagnoses	☐	☐	☐	☐

Behavioural objectives: management

	N/A	Not Done	Done: needs improvement	Done: meets expectations
Determine appropriate treatment environment: inpatient vs. outpatient	☐	☐	☐	☐
If patient has harmed self: address medical complications	☐	☐	☐	☐
Address access to means of suicide	☐	☐	☐	☐
Enlist support systems, such as family members	☐	☐	☐	☐
Address comorbid substance use	☐	☐	☐	☐
Address medical problems and medications, including ordering lab tests	☐	☐	☐	☐
Use appropriate Rx for depression, anxiety or insomnia	☐	☐	☐	☐
Provide patient with contact information	☐	☐	☐	☐
Discuss treatment plan with patient using non-technical language	☐	☐	☐	☐
Work collaboratively with patient, instilling hope	☐	☐	☐	☐
Work as a team with faculty, first-year resident, ED staff	☐	☐	☐	☐

APPENDIX 8.3 ASSESSMENT FORM FOR 'ACUTE PSYCHOSIS'

University of Wisconsin Psychiatry Residency
Evaluation of Basic Emergency Psychiatry Skills (Accompanied Call)
ACUTE PSYCHOSIS OR MANIA

Resident:_____   Date:_____

Attending:_____

Behavioural objectives: assessment	N/A	Not Done	Done: needs improvement	Done: meets expectations
Culturally sensitive and empathic	☐	☐	☐	☐
Establishes and maintains rapport	☐	☐	☐	☐
Focused and efficient interview	☐	☐	☐	☐
Psychotic symptoms, including positive and negative	☐	☐	☐	☐
Symptoms of mania and depression	☐	☐	☐	☐
Psychiatric sx: anxiety, substance use, suicidality, homicidality	☐	☐	☐	☐
Recent psychosocial stressors and precipitants	☐	☐	☐	☐
Support systems	☐	☐	☐	☐
Past psychiatric history, including review of medical records	☐	☐	☐	☐
Concurrent medical problems and medication use	☐	☐	☐	☐
Relevant developmental history	☐	☐	☐	☐
Physical exam, lab work and imaging	☐	☐	☐	☐
MSE, especially cognition (orientation, attention, memory)	☐	☐	☐	☐
Collateral information to corroborate history	☐	☐	☐	☐
Preliminary biopsychosocial formulation and DSM-IV axial diagnoses	☐	☐	☐	☐

Behavioural objectives: management	N/A	Not Done	Done: needs improvement	Done: meets expectations
Determine appropriate treatment environment: inpatient medical, inpatient psychiatric or outpatient	☐	☐	☐	☐
Address medical problems & medications, including ordering lab tests and imaging	☐	☐	☐	☐
Address comorbid substance use	☐	☐	☐	☐
Enlist support systems, such as family members	☐	☐	☐	☐
Use appropriate Rx for psychosis, mania, agitation or insomnia	☐	☐	☐	☐
Provide patient with contact information	☐	☐	☐	☐
Discuss treatment plan with patient using non-technical language	☐	☐	☐	☐
Work collaboratively with patient, instilling hope	☐	☐	☐	☐
Work as a team with faculty, first-year resident, ED staff	☐	☐	☐	☐

APPENDIX 8.4 ASSESSMENT FORM FOR 'SUBSTANCE INTOXICATION'

University of Wisconsin Psychiatry Residency
Evaluation of Basic Emergency Psychiatry Skills (Accompanied Call)
SUBSTANCE INTOXICATION OR WITHDRAWAL

Resident:_____   Date:_____

Attending:_____

Behavioural objectives: assessment	N/A	Not Done	Done: needs improvement	Done: meets expectations
Culturally sensitive and empathic	☐	☐	☐	☐
Establishes and maintains rapport	☐	☐	☐	☐
Focused and efficient interview	☐	☐	☐	☐
Classes of substances: alcohol, sedative-hypnotics, opioids, stimulants, hallucinogens, cannabis	☐	☐	☐	☐
Pattern of use: amount, frequency of use, time last used	☐	☐	☐	☐
Classic symptoms of intoxication and withdrawal	☐	☐	☐	☐
Psychiatric sx: depression, anxiety, mania, psychosis, suicidality, homicidality, aggression	☐	☐	☐	☐
Recent psychosocial stressors and precipitants	☐	☐	☐	☐
Support systems	☐	☐	☐	☐
Past psychiatric history, including review of medical records	☐	☐	☐	☐
Concurrent medical problems and medication use	☐	☐	☐	☐
Relevant developmental history	☐	☐	☐	☐
Physical examination and lab work	☐	☐	☐	☐
MSE, especially cognition (orientation, attention, memory)	☐	☐	☐	☐
Collateral information to corroborate history	☐	☐	☐	☐
Preliminary biopsychosocial formulation & DSM-IV axial diagnoses	☐	☐	☐	☐

Behavioural objectives: management	N/A	Not Done	Done: needs improvement	Done: meets expectations
Determine appropriate treatment environment: inpatient medical, inpatient psychiatric or outpatient	☐	☐	☐	☐
Address medical problems & medications, including ordering lab tests	☐	☐	☐	☐
Anticipate/manage alcohol, benzo or opioid withdrawal	☐	☐	☐	☐
Enlist support systems, such as family members	☐	☐	☐	☐
Address anxiety, insomnia or agitation	☐	☐	☐	☐
Provide patient with contact information	☐	☐	☐	☐
Discuss treatment plan with patient using non-technical language	☐	☐	☐	☐
Work collaboratively with patient, instilling hope	☐	☐	☐	☐
Work as a team with faculty, first-year resident, ED staff	☐	☐	☐	☐

REFERENCES

AADPRT (2010a). *Mission Statement.* http://www.aadprt.org/pages.aspx?PageName= Mission_Statement.

AADPRT (2010b). *A Reflection on the History of AADPRT.* http://www.aadprt.org/pages. aspx?PageName=AADPRT_History).

ACGME (2000). *Toolbox of Assessment Methods.* http://www.acgme.org/outcome/assess/ toolbox.asp.

ACGME (2005). *The ACGME Outcome Project: An Introduction.* http://www.acgme.org/ Outcome/.

Philibert, I., Johnston, M. J., Hruska, L. *et al.* (2010). Institutional attributes associated with innovation and improvement: results of a multisite study. *Journal of Graduate Medical Education,* **2**(2), 306–312.

Satish, U., Manring, J., Gregory, R. *et al.* (2009). Novel assessments of psychiatry residents: SMS simulations. *ACGME Bulletin,* (January), 18–23. http://www.acgme. org/acWebsite/bulletin/bulletin0109.pdf.

West, C. P., Huntington, J. L., Huschka, M. M. *et al.* (2007). A prospective study of the relationship between medical knowledge and professionalism among internal medicine residents. *Academic Medicine,* **82**(6), 587–592.

9

The Australian and New Zealand experience

Christine Spratt, Philip Boyce and Mark Davies

Editors' introduction

This chapter by Christine Spratt and colleagues from Australia and New Zealand outlines the manner in which the profession in these two countries has been proactive in responding both to the socio-political climate and to international developments in postgraduate medical education by taking the lead in trying to transform postgraduate psychiatric training in Australia and New Zealand. The financial support of this process by the Australian Federal Government sets a commendable benchmark for other statutory organizations across the world. The developments within postgraduate psychiatric training in these two countries are also remarkable, as those leading the change have gone to great lengths to draw on and learn from the wider international experience in this area. The chapter details the efforts of the Curriculum Improvement Project (CIP) to define the process of development and create different stages of training. It also describes the utility of Entrustable Professional Activities (EPAs) in relation to the CanMEDS Framework to support the development of competent performance for trainees in Australia and New Zealand.

Introduction

This chapter describes the recent experience of the Royal Australian and New Zealand College of Psychiatrists (the College) in implementing workplace-based assessment as part of an extensive curriculum reform project. The chapter first describes the context for change in specialist training in psychiatry in Australia and New Zealand. It briefly reviews the imperatives for the adoption of an outcome-based curriculum model and describes the College's approach to the adoption and

Workplace-Based Assessments in Psychiatric Training, ed. Dinesh Bhugra and Amit Malik.
Published by Cambridge University Press. © Cambridge University Press 2011.

implementation of the CanMEDS framework. It proceeds to illustrate the way in which the integration of performance or workplace-based assessment will occur across the Fellowship programme.

The context for change at the RANZCP

In the past two decades the healthcare environment has come under considerable pressure in Australia and internationally, not least from increased demand, workforce shortages in all medical specialties and changing work practices (Afrin *et al.*, 2006; AHMAC, 2002; Dowton, 2005; Medical Specialist Training Steering Committee, 2006), reflecting the urgent need for sustainable workforce planning.

These trends internationally have led to changes in curricula from more traditional apprenticeship models to those that reflect competency or outcome-based educational frameworks (Dowton, 2005; Faught, 2004; Frank and Danoff, 2007; Frieman *et al.*, 2006). In some medical education jurisdictions this is demonstrated by dramatic changes in the governance of postgraduate medical education, for example, in the United States (ACGME, 2005), the Netherlands (Scheele *et al.*, 2008), Canada (Frank and Danoff, 2007; RCPSC, 2007) and, most recently, the United Kingdom (MMC, 2007; PMETB, 2007), as related governing bodies respond to pressures for educational change. Given these matters, the College has chosen to be proactive and review its broad educational values and the educational framework that underpins its curriculum.

The College's decision to look more critically at its educational and assessment practices has been supported by an extensive five-year Curriculum Improvement Project (CIP) funded in part by the Australian Federal Government. The CIP is principally concerned with curriculum renewal and redevelopment of the existing RANZCP five-year Fellowship training programme. In the contemporary postgraduate educational environment this necessarily calls for more determined measures of performance in 'authentic' settings (Challis, 2005; Herrington and Herrington, 2006) and in medical education this is now commonly seen in moves towards competency or outcome-based curricula and the integration of workplace-based assessment in specialist training (Jolly, 2007; Norcini 2003; Schuwirth and van der Vleuten, 2006a; Bhugra *et al.*, 2007).

The College's existing curriculum is based on a broad bio-psycho-socio-cultural model and realized through the principles of apprenticeship, where learning is supported by expert supervision and a formal education course. The current Fellowship training programme consists of a minimum of three years basic training (BT), followed by a minimum of two years advanced training (AT) in an approved programme of advanced training or the generalist stream following completion of summative assessment (an OSCE and observed clinical interview (OCI)). Basic training directs trainees through a number of mandatory rotations (adult; child and adolescent; consultation liaison) and mandatory experiences (non-government organization; consumer; carer; Aboriginal and Torres Strait Islanders and Maori) and approved training (old age, addiction, psychotherapy, ECT), punctuated with supervisor and summative assessments including two case history submissions, a written examination and two mid-point clinical examinations (OSCE and OCI). While the curriculum is largely experiential, trainees are also required to complete concurrently a formal education course (FEC), which addresses the academic psychiatry syllabus.

Advanced training allows trainees to enter into either a generalist stream or an approved programme (forensic; adult; psychotherapies; old age; child and adolescent; addiction; consultation liaison) or a combination of the two. Seven core advanced training experiences must also be completed (management in psychological, biological, social, cultural aspects in psychiatry; consultative skills; CME activities; leadership and management skills and a completed psychotherapy case). The apprenticeship model is maintained in advanced training; however the emphasis is placed on self-directed learning.

Despite the temporal aspect of training being somewhat antithetical to the principles understood to underpin competency-based education, the changes implemented by the College will necessarily be practically constrained by time to some degree, owing to the allocation and rotation of trainees through training posts in health jurisdictions. These organizational structures force us into a compromise position.

It is important to note that training in Australia and New Zealand is undertaken predominately in the public sector, where there is a rapid turnover of high-acuity patients with psychosis; furthermore service demands create a challenging environment for trainees that often allows limited opportunities for reflective learning.

Given this, the current curriculum is effectively a distributed educational programme managed centrally but implemented and taught locally by a complex integrated system of local training committees in health jurisdictions. Regional programmes are managed by Directors of Training. The characteristic feature of the current programme is its heavy reliance on the goodwill of consultant psychiatrists who provide largely pro-bono supervision of trainees and who cooperate and collaborate with their Directors of Training to assure the programme's standards.

The CanMEDS framework for the RANZCP

The College believes that the curriculum ought to be informed by a more *effective* and *efficient* outcome-oriented framework than is currently the case and that it should better reflect the College's commitment to *continuous improvement* as 'fit-for-purpose' in its educational undertakings. Like other apprenticeship models, the College's current programme has been subject to criticism internally and from its accreditor, the Australian Medical Council (AMC). Specifically, in the recent past, AMC reviews highlighted that the College's programme reflected:

• Poor curriculum alignment between stated learning objectives, teaching and learning strategies and assessment requirements;

- Perceived variability in the quality of the FEC, which currently ranges from a Master's qualification in one state to locally coordinated programmes in other state and territory jurisdictions;
- Competing demands for service provision and training requirements for trainees; and
- Extended time taken for trainees to complete the programme.

Consequently the College's governing body, the General Council, approved the decision to adopt the highly regarded CanMEDS framework produced by the Royal College of Physicians and Surgeons of Canada (RCPSC, 2007) to underpin its curriculum renewal.

The CanMEDS framework preceded by a decade other developing frameworks, in particular 'The Outcome Project' of the American Graduate Council for Medical Education and the 'Modernising Medical Careers' initiative in the United Kingdom (UK). This accounts for the highly influential role that CanMEDS has played in informing global movements in postgraduate medical education. More recently, the RCPSC has collaborated with specific medical specialty groups across Canada to design specialty-specific models and the Specialist Committee in Psychiatry developed its 'Objectives for Training in Psychiatry', which extends the more generic CanMEDS roles to psychiatry. The psychiatry objectives marry the CanMEDS framework with more specific training objectives that aim to guide the design of the particular psychiatry training 'path' or learning programme.

We believe that CanMEDS supports a more holistic and qualitative approach to competence, which better reflects the contemporary professional practice than behavioural or 'skills-based' approaches to competence. We have attempted to define this more qualitative approach as 'competent performance' and have drawn on Govaerts (2008) and McAllister (2005) to inform our thinking. Graduate outcomes will be explicitly informed by the concept of 'competent performance' where:

Competent performance refers to the capable exercise of professional judgment in practice settings of change and impermanence; it is always developmental and context dependent. Competent performance implies the integration of knowledge, skills, judgment and attitudes. Competent performance is linked to professional roles and domains of practice and demands self-regulation and critical reflection.

Medical practice does not occur in isolation; we need to work with and communicate effectively with carers and consumers in ways that are made explicit in the CanMEDS model. Curricula that have an explicit focus on the roles of carers, the patient or consumer and multi-disciplinary colleagues, must prepare specialist clinicians to practise in accordance with the expectations of stakeholders and the edicts of their profession. Competent performance is therefore particularly relevant to the important and complex roles and responsibilities held by psychiatrists within mental health systems and the community more generally.

A programme approach to assessment

It is now widely accepted across the post-secondary sector that assessment drives learning – it is neither peripheral nor additional and it is most beneficial when it is ongoing (formative) rather than episodic. It should be reflected across the curriculum as multi-dimensional, integrated, authentic and performance-based. Models of assessment should foster learning *and* measure learning outcomes; that is, assessment *for* learning and assessment *of* learning (Carless, 2007); assessment strategies should be authentic, valid and reliable. An aligned system of learning is imperative to success and demands that learning outcomes (or competencies), teaching strategies and assessment approaches are coherent and integrated, thereby offering assurances to stakeholders that graduates – in our case specialist psychiatrists – meet desired performance outcomes (Biggs and Tang, 2007; Shumway and Harden, 2003; Carless, 2007).

We are therefore committed to developing a more transparent programme approach to assessment. This is in keeping with contemporary approaches to curriculum alignment evident in the higher education sector (Biggs and Tang, 2007; Boud and Falchikov, 2006; James, 2002; Nicol, 2007) and growing calls for such approaches in specialist medical education (Grant, 2007; PMETB, 2007; Schuwirth and van der Vleuten, 2004; 2006b).

One stage of our assessment framework is the identification of the developmental trajectory that we will use to define the progress of competence at the major points on our curriculum. Table 9.1 illustrates the trajectory for the early years of training (currently Years 1–3). Table 9.2 identifies the trajectory for the stages that we are defining as 'advanced competency', using child and adolescent psychiatry as an exemplar. The developmental trajectory will assist us in determining performance and assessment standards.

Assessing competent performance

Workplace-based assessment (or in-training assessment) is an integral part of a competency-based curriculum. It refers to those formative and summative strategies that attempt to measure performance in authentic settings in the workplace; importantly, such assessment should be developed to provide an objective and transparent measure of the doctors' capabilities in practice (Archer *et al.*, 2006; Bhugra *et al.*, 2007; Brown and Doshi, 2006; Carraccio and Englander, 2004; Veloski *et al.*, 2006). There is an increasing amount of literature on the subject across the medical education sector and while debates regarding the validity and reliability of various forms of workplace-based assessment have yet to reach consensus (Murphy *et al.*, 2009; Norcini and Burch, 2007), there is substantial preliminary evidence to inform approaches to guide assessment practices (Bhugra *et al.*, 2007; Grant, 2007; Murphy *et al.*, 2009; Ringsted *et al.*, 2004; Schuwirth and van der Vleuten, 2004; van der Vleuten and Schuwirth, 2005).

Table 9.1 Developmental trajectory (early years)

Novice	Basic	Proficient
Trainee has the ability to recognize, identify and describe the core principles of psychiatry, including introductory knowledge of high-prevalence conditions and emergency presentations	Trainee is able to demonstrate core aspects of psychiatry, such as basic interviewing, problem formulation and treatment. Trainee demonstrates working knowledge of psychiatry, including understanding of the scientific literature and the ability to interpret the clinical findings in high-prevalence conditions and emergency presentations	Trainee demonstrates basic knowledge enhanced by a developmental, cultural and lifespan perspective, allowing detailed interviewing and biopsychosocial problem formulation with the capacity to teach, consult, assess and manage referrals
Trainee relies on linear thinking and pattern recognition to make decisions		Trainee shows evidence of a shift in thinking from linear relationships to more holistic interpretations of clinical problems
Trainee's perception of the situation is largely informed by abstract principles and theoretical concepts	The trainee has moved from a reliance on abstract principles to the use of past concrete experience to inform decision-making	Proficiency defines personal qualities and specialist expertise developed through critical self-reflection and the application of specialist knowledge and skills. This reflects the ability to apply evidence-based practice, peer review and recognitions of the need for ongoing supervision
Trainee requires supervision while developing skill in the areas of formulation, intervention and management planning	Trainee can accurately assess the presenting complexity and describe a rationale for decision-making	
Trainee demonstrates awareness of evidence-based practice and is able to apply evidence-based treatment approaches to familiar presentations with support	In high-prevalence conditions and emergency presentations, trainee can accurately communicate clinical findings to patients, families and carers	

Table 9.2 Advanced competency trajectory, example of child and adolescent psychiatry

Entry: specialty	Advanced	Exit (consultant)
Will require assistance to recognize the level of complexity in their work	Accurately assess the level of complexity and identify the rationale for their judgement	Accurately address complex clinical and systems issues independently and efficiently
Undertake any aspect of work with regular supervision and support	Undertakes routine or familiar work independently and seek supervision to manage complex or novel work	Able to manage complex or novel work but seek supervision and support where the circumstances require it
Demonstrate basic knowledge relevant to child and adolescent psychiatry and require support and supervision to apply these to practice	Able to actively apply current knowledge and skills, and address gaps with support	Able to integrate and apply new knowledge and recognize gaps in knowledge and apply to current practice

| Low independence | Moderate independence | High independence |

Entrustable professional activities, performance assessment and CanMEDS

The College's proposed approach to workplace-based assessment has been heavily informed by work from the United Kingdom on assessment generally (PMETB, 2007), work specifically on the assessment of psychiatry (Bhugra *et al.*, 2007; Stubbe *et al.*, 2007) and the Canadian experience (Frank and Danoff, 2007; RCPSC, 2007). More recently, the latest work from Olle ten Cate's group in the Netherlands (ten Cate, 2005; ten Cate and Scheele, 2007) has been influential in assisting us to conceive how we might address some of the more conceptual issues emerging from CanMEDS and the assessment of competent performance.

Furthermore, as we work towards the integration of the CanMEDS roles and competency standards in our curriculum, we aim to assure that we do not atomize skills such that 'incompetence' is encouraged (Hodges, 2006). Key knowledge, skills and attitudes, the traditional informants of curricula, are best incorporated with competence development in an integrated manner such that performance outcomes are assessed in the real world of clinical practice and that activities that are to be assessed are regularly practised.

While the integration of CanMEDS in the existing curriculum poses considerable challenges, we are mindful that we must adopt innovative strategies that will generate valid, reliable assessments that are relevant for our complex environment and that reflect best practice internationally in the emerging literature. As we have already described, the Fellowship programme is delivered binationally in a complex health and socio-political environment. This section outlines the key pragmatic considerations that the College faces in designing and implementing workplace-based assessment.

As indicated, we have found ten Cate's 2005 concept of entrustable professional activities (EPA) a useful tool to determine the way in which the CanMEDS roles can best be integrated into our existing curriculum and establish a workplace-based assessment system. Following from this, ten Cate's group developed three key criteria (ten Cate and Scheele, 2007) to identify an entrustable professional activity:
1. A task of high importance for daily practice (core business);
2. A high-risk or error-prone task; and
3. A task that is exemplary for (a number of) specific CanMEDS roles.

For ten Cate, an entrustable professional activity is 'a unit of work that should be only entrusted upon a competent enough professional' (ten Cate and Scheele, 2007, p. 544). Essentially then, entrustable professional activities can be used to map to the CanMEDS roles and competencies and therefore to *infer* the development of competence.

Entrustable professional activities are identified by disciplinary experts as an essential part of work in any given context, so present an opportune and authentic means of quantifying professional disciplinary knowledge and performances. They have the potential to identify when trainees can be 'entrusted' to progress to increasingly sophisticated levels of independence; for us, this means progression along our identified developmental trajectory so that the trainee requires diminishing levels of supervision; that is, becomes increasingly independent. Entrustable professional activities can be quite conveniently aligned to broad and specific learning objectives and mapped to various competency standards; in our case, to the seven CanMEDS roles and their specific standard statements.

As part of our developing workplace-based assessment models, the CIP is defining the competencies and standards to which they need to be achieved in basic training aligned to CanMEDS. As part of this development, we surveyed Fellows to identify clinical activities that a trainee in Year 1, for example, should be able to carry out independently (with minimal supervision, or at least recognizing where additional supervision is required) to assist us identify our own EPAs. In our case, 480 responses were received to an email invitation to all Fellows ($n = 3000$) to participate in the survey, a response rate of 16%. Results indicated high levels of consensus on the activities identified as mandatory for trainees to demonstrate competency prior to sub-specialty training. This was particularly true in the core medical features of psychiatry, including initiating a patient on medication, admitting and discharging a patient, and assessment. The results were more variable in the area of family education sessions and the provision of psychotherapy, with qualitative comments indicating that these are skills that develop over the course of the training programme. Areas that were identified as necessary for

Entrustable professional activities [EPAs]: Year 1 (CIP 300609)

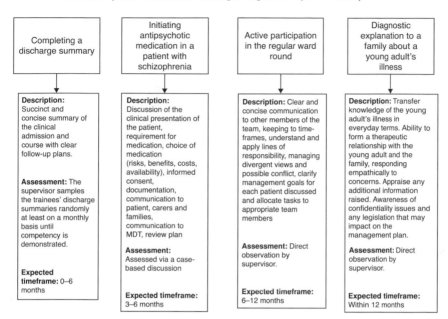

Figure 9.1 Proposed RANZCP EPAs for Year 1

inclusion in proposed EPAs were greater emphasis on medico-legal issues, including the role of guardianship and reporting requirements in relation to children and families. Qualitative data also indicated that consideration of an EPA relating to communication, particularly with colleagues and supervisors, would also be important.

From this survey and other internal consultations, and subsequent to confirmation by the CIP Reference Committee, we have identified four major EPAs that characterize Year 1 (see Figure 9.1). We have used these EPAs over the past six months in various working parties as we move to establish competencies, standards, learning experiences and a potential assessment strategy for Year 1. To accommodate the variety in experiences across training programmes, we anticipate extending the provisional number of EPAs to six or eight to allow supervisors and directors of training some scope and flexibility in the use of EPAs to design and direct learning experiences.

As we envisage the curriculum, trainees would have to demonstrate that they can perform EPAs before they can progress to the sub-specialty rotations. The identified EPAs have been aligned to the relevant CanMEDS roles and a mapping or blueprinting matrix developed as part of the developing curriculum design. There has been considerable interest in this strategy across the College's education portfolio. Anecdotally, our expert working groups see considerable potential in continuing to refine and identify EPAs. Based on the preliminary survey data and the views of such groups, the CIP Reference Committee aims to use the EPAs to rationalize for our stakeholders, especially supervisors, the rather conceptual nature of CanMEDS into a more transparent and pragmatic curriculum. This is in keeping with emerging strategies and data presented by Scheele and ten Cate and their colleagues (Dijksterhuis *et al.*, 2009).

Once the EPAs are identified, we believe that we will be better able to structure a clear, transparent and well-aligned formative assessment programme. Each EPA can therefore be 'unpacked' to reflect the underlying competencies and also assist us to identify trainees who may be demonstrating difficulties and who may need focused remediation. Given our current approach, we anticipate that the assessment programme will draw on the kinds of workplace-based assessment that are currently being implemented across the sector.

In particular, we are interested in case-based discussion, multi-source feedback and the mini-CEX (or mini-ACE). We expect to see changes in the way in which our current summative observed clinical interview (OCI) is used. In our new system, the OCI will be formative and in–training rather than a high-stake 'one-off' summative assessment integrated with the current clinical OSCE. Given our use of CanMEDS, we are also interested in the way that the Royal College of Physicians and Surgeons of Canada approaches summative in-training assessment. One of the compelling arguments for competency-based medical education and workplace-based assessment, aside from better measures of performance, lies in the way in which timely and appropriate feedback to trainees can be integrated more explicitly with authentic assessment. The proposed changes to the curriculum and assessment models potentially allow for more rigorous and transparent feedback processes than exist within the current programme. The planned workplace-based assessment models will be more explicitly aligned to expected outcomes and have greater potential to allow for the provision of more appropriate feedback and for the development of trainees' capacity for critical self-reflection and to assess their own stage of learning and competence development (Chur-Hansen and McLean, 2006; Combs *et al.*, 2008; Daelmans *et al.*, 2006). Figure 9.2 illustrates the development model.

Conclusion

The College accepts that postgraduate medical education must prepare specialist psychiatrists who are creative problem-solvers – critical thinkers capable of innovative practice and committed to accepted professional and societal standards of patient-centred care. The Fellowship curriculum must be informed by defensible educational approaches that promote self-regulation and responsibility for one's own professional development across the lifetime of professional practice.

This chapter has described how we believe the CanMEDS framework will allow us to develop our curriculum strategically against an internationally accepted benchmark. Further, we believe that it will enable us to design an assessment

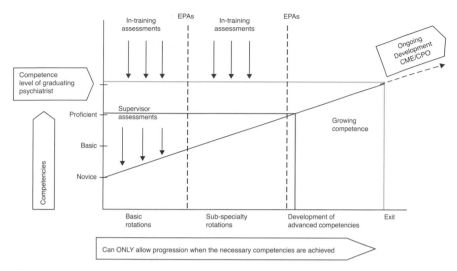

Figure 9.2 CanMEDS, EPAs and developing competent performance in the RANZCP Fellowship Programme

programme that is well-aligned to the identified outcome standards, which will satisfy all stakeholders that workplace based assessments can be designed and demonstrated to be valid, and reliable measures of the competent performance of the specialist psychiatrist. The workplace-based assessment model that we will implement in the next year or two will be the focus of determined review and evaluation, in particular, in relation to assessing the potential that we have identified in this chapter for the use of EPAs in assisting to define the CanMEDS competencies in practice and in designing the assessment of the CanMEDS roles and competencies.

REFERENCES

ACGME (2005). *The ACGME Outcome Project: An Introduction.* http://www.acgme.org/Outcome/.

Afrin, L. B., Arana, G. W., Medio, F. J., Ybarra, A. F. and Clarke, H. S. (2006). Improving oversight of the graduate medical education enterprise: one institution's strategies and tools. *Academic Medicine*, **81**(5), 419–425.

Archer, J., Norcini, J., Southgate, L., Heard, S. and Davies, H. (2006). Mini-PAT (peer assessment tool): a valid component of a national assessment programme in the UK? *Advances in Health Sciences Education Theory and Practice*, **13**, 181–192.

AHMAC (Australian Health Ministers' Advisory Council) (2002). *Medical Specialist Education and Training: Responding to the Impact of Changes in Australia's Health Care System. A Discussion Paper.* Melbourne. http://www.health.gov.au/internet/main/publishing.nsf/Content/work-edu-spectr-respond.

Bhugra, D., Malik, A. and Brown, N. (2007). *Workplace-Based Assessments in Psychiatry*, London: Royal College of Psychiatry Publications.

Biggs, J. and Tang, C. (2007). *Teaching for Quality Learning at University*, 3rd edn. Buckingham, SRHE and Open University Press.

Boud, D. and Falchikov, N. (2006). Aligning assessment with long-term learning. *Assessment and Evaluation in Higher Education*, **31**(4), 399–413.

Brown, N. and Doshi, M. (2006). Assessing professional and clinical competence: the way forward. *Advances in Psychiatric Treatment*, **12**, 81–91.

Carless, D. (2007). Learning-oriented assessment: conceptual bases and practical implications. *Innovations in Education and Teaching International*, **44**(1) 57–66.

Carraccio, C. and Englander, R. (2004). Evaluating competence using a portfolio: a literature review and web-based application to the ACGME competencies. *Teaching and Learning in Medicine*, **16**(4), 381–387.

Challis, D. (2005). Committing to quality learning through adaptive online assessment. *Assessment and Evaluation in Higher Education*, **30**(5), 519–527.

Chur-Hansen, A. and McLean, S. (2006). On being a supervisor: the importance of feedback and how to give it. *Australasian Psychiatry*, **14**(1), 67–71.

Combs, K. L., Gibson, S. K., Hays, J. M., Saly, J. and Wendt, J. T. (2008). Enhancing curriculum and delivery: linking assessment to learning objectives. *Assessment and Evaluation in Higher Education*, **33**(1), 87–102.

Daelmans, H., Overmeer, R., van der Hem-Stokroos, H. *et al.* (2006). In-training assessment: qualitative study of effects on supervision and feedback in an undergraduate clinical rotation. *Medical Education*, **40**(1), 51–58.

Dijksterhuis, M., Voorhuis, M., Teunissen, P. *et al.* (2009). Assessment of competence and progressive independence in postgraduate clinical training, *Medical Education*, **43**, 1156–1165.

Dowton, B. (2005). Imperatives in medical education and training in response to demands for a sustainable workforce. *Medical Journal of Australia*, **183**, (11/12), 595–598.

Faught, W. (2004). CanMEDs roles and obstetrics and gynaecology: the time is now. *Journal of Obstetrics and Gynaecology Canada*, **26**(9), 781–784.

Frank, J. R. and Danoff, D. (2007). The CanMEDS initiative: implementing an outcomes-based framework of physician competencies. *Medical Teacher*, **29**(7), 642–647.

Frieman, A., Natesh, A., Barankin, B. and Shear, N. (2006). Dermatology postgraduate training in Canada: CanMEDS competencies. *Dermatology Online*, **12**(1), 6.

Govaerts, M. J. B. (2008). Educational competencies or education for professional competence? *Medical Education*, **42**(3), 234–236.

Grant, J. (2007). Changing postgraduate medical education: a commentary from the United Kingdom. *Medical Journal of Australia*, **186**, 7(Supplement), S9–S13.

Herrington, A. and Herrington, J. (2006). *Authentic Learning Environments in Higher Education*. London: Idea Group.

Hodges, B. (2006). Medical education and the maintenance of incompetence. *Medical Teacher*, **28**(8), 690–696.

James, R. (2002). *Assessing Learning in Australian Universities*, http://www.cshe.unimelb.edu.au/assessinglearning/index.html.

Jolly, B. (2007). The new curriculum framework and assessment practices: current challenges for postgraduate years 1 and 2. *Medical Journal of Australia*, **186**(7), S33–S36.

McAllister, S. (2005). *Competency Based Assessment of Speech Pathology Students' Performance in the Workplace*, Ph.D. thesis, Sydney: School of Communication Sciences and Disorders, University of Sydney.

Medical Specialist Training Steering Committee (2006). *More Doctors, Better Training: Specialist Medical Training to Meet the Needs of All Australians to 2016.* Reference Group 3 Report. Canberra: Department of Health and Ageing. http://www.health.gov.au/internet/main/publishing.nsf/Content/work-edu-spectr-mstsc-rept-toc~work-edu-spectr-mstsc-rept-app-e.

MMC (Modernising Medical Careers) (2007). *A Guide to Postgraduate Specialty Training in the UK: The Gold Guide.* http://www.mmc.nhs.uk/pdf/Gold%20Guide%202007.pdf.

Murphy, D. J., Bruce, D. A., Mercer, S. W. and Eva, K. W. (2009). The reliability of workplace-based assessment in postgraduate medical education and training: a national evaluation in general practice in the United Kingdom. *Advances in Health Sciences Education Theory Practice*, **14**(2), 219–232.

Nicol, D. (2007). Principles of good assessment and feedback: Theory and practice. *From the REAP International Online Conference on Assessment Design for Learner Responsibility, 29th–31st May 2007.* http://www.reap.ac.uk/public/Papers/Principles_of_good_assessment_and_feedback.pdf; http://www.reap.ac.uk/resources.html.

Norcini, J. (2003). ABC of learning and teaching in medicine; work based assessment. *BMJ*, **326**, 753–755.

Norcini, J. and Burch, V. (2007). Workplace-based assessment as an educational tool: AMEE Guide No 31. *Medical Teacher*, **29**(9), 855–871.

PMETB (Postgraduate Medical Education and Training Board) (2007). *Developing and Maintaining an Assessment System – A PMETB Guide to Good Practice*, Postgraduate Medical Education and Training Board. http://www.gmc-uk.org/Assessment_good_practice_v0207.pdf_31385949.pdf.

RCPSC (Royal College of Physicians and Surgeons of Canada) (2007). *The CanMEDS Framework.* http://rcpsc.medical.org/canmeds/.

Ringsted, C., Henriksen, A. H., Skaarup, A. M. and van der Vleuten, C. P. (2004). Educational impact of in-training assessment (ITA) in postgraduate medical education: a qualitative study of an ITA programme in actual practice. *Medical Education*, **38**(7), 767–777.

Scheele, F., Teunissen, P., van Luijk, S. *et al.* (2008). Introducing competency-based postgraduate medical education in the Netherlands. *Medical Teacher*, **30**(3), 248–253.

Schuwirth, L. W. T. and van der Vleuten, C. P. M. (2004). Changing education, changing assessment, changing research? *Medical Education*, **38**(8), 805–812.

Schuwirth, L. W. T. and van der Vleuten, C.P. (2006a). Challenges for educationalists. *BMJ*, **333**, 7657.

Schuwirth, L. W. and van der Vleuten, C. P. (2006b). A plea for new psychometric models in educational assessment. *Medical Education*, **40**(4), 296–300.

Shumway, J. M. and Harden, R. M. (2003). AMEE Guide No. 25: The assessment of learning outcomes for the competent and reflective physician. *Medical Teacher*, **25**(6), 569–584.

Stubbe, D., Heyneman, E. and Stock, S. (2007). A stitch in time saves nine: intervention strategies for the remediation of competency. *Child and Adolescent Psychiatric Clinics of North America*, **16**(1), 249–264.

ten Cate, O. (2005). Entrustability of professional activities and competency based training. *Medical Education*, **39**, 1176–1177.

ten Cate, O. and Scheele, F. (2007). Competency-based postgraduate training: Can we bridge the gap between theory and clinical practice? *Academic Medicine*, **82**, 542–547.

van der Vleuten, C. and Schuwirth, L. (2005). Assessing professional competence: from methods to programmes. *Medical Education*, **39**(3), 309–317.

Veloski, J., Boex, J. R., Grasberger, M. J., Evans, A. and Wolfson, D. B. (2006). Systematic review of the literature on assessment, feedback and physician's clinical performance: BEME Guide No 7. *Medical Teacher*, **28**(2), 117–128.

10

The Canadian experience

Karen Saperson and Richard P. Swinson

Editors' introduction

The CanMEDS 2000 project, which was innovated and developed in Canada, was ground-breaking in terms of developing a physician competency framework, and Canada was one of the first countries to adopt it within postgraduate psychiatric training in the last decade. Whilst outlining changes in postgraduate assessments and evaluation in psychiatry in Canada over the last decade, this chapter also gives an interesting account of how the national move from the long case assessment to the Objective Structured Clinical Examination (OSCE), as a result of concerns regarding the reliability of the long case assessment, led to anxieties amongst senior educators nationally regarding the validity and the educational impact of only using the OSCE for assessments. This highlights once again the importance of the programmatic approach to the development of assessment tools and the need for compromises within different aspects of utility to meet the overall purpose of the assessment framework. Interestingly, the significant concerns about only using a national-level OSCE led to the development of the STACER (standardized assessment of a clinical encounter report), highlighting again the importance of attaining a balance between formative local assessment and summative national assessments that are not only valid and reliable, but also have the desired educational impact. These developments in Canada have not been without their challenges and they are also discussed here. The chapter also provides some insight into a unique programme for training and assessing international medical graduates, who form a significant proportion of the psychiatric workforce, especially in the Western world.

Workplace-Based Assessments in Psychiatric Training, ed. Dinesh Bhugra and Amit Malik. Published by Cambridge University Press. © Cambridge University Press 2011.

Introduction

Psychiatry in Canada was first recognized as a medical specialty in the division of specialties in 1944 and the first psychiatrists were awarded certificates in 1946. The history of the development of Canadian psychiatry has been ably documented by Rae-Grant (Rae-Grant, 1996). The history and background of developments in psychiatric training are described by Swinson and Leverette (2009) in *Approaches to Postgraduate Education in Psychiatry in Canada*, published by the Canadian Psychiatric Association. The Royal College of Physicians and Surgeons of Canada oversees the medical education of specialists in Canada. The office of education of the College sets the standards for postgraduate medical education, accredits specialty residency programmes and is responsible for conducting certifying examinations (RCPSC, 2009a).

CanMEDS

The CanMEDS physician competency framework was adopted by the Royal College in 1996 and significantly updated in 2005 (Frank, 2005). This innovative framework for medical education evolved out of the CanMEDS 2000 project, which was commissioned in 1993 to examine societal healthcare needs in Canada and to assess the implications for postgraduate specialty training programmes.

The project embodies two fundamental concepts;
1. Changing the focus of specialty training from the interests and abilities of providers to the needs of society, and
2. Orienting these programmes to consider the needs of individual patients in context of the population at large.

(Frank *et al.*, 1996).

The resulting framework describes seven major roles, with the medical expert role playing a central role and the roles of communicator, collaborator, manager, health advocate, scholar and professional overlapping and equally important.

The CanMEDS competencies have been integrated into the Royal College's accreditation standards, objectives of training, final in-training evaluations, examination blueprints and the maintenance of certification programme.

The CanMEDS diagram (Figure 10.1) was created to illustrate these elements and is known as the CanMEDS 'cloverleaf' or 'daisy'. (RCPSC, 2007a)

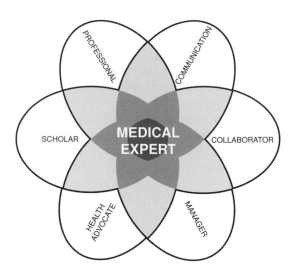

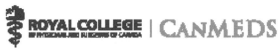

Figure 10.1 The 'daisy' design illustrates the CanMEDS framework. © 2003 Royal College of Physicians and Surgeons of Canada.

Description of current training with emphasis on 2007 changes

Residency training in psychiatry in Canada has undergone significant changes in the past decade. The evolution of these changes (detailed in the Royal College of Physician and Surgeons Objectives of Training (OTR) and Specialty Training Requirements (STR) for Psychiatry), has been well-documented (Leverette, 2009). A number of significant revisions have been made to the OTR and STR even within the last two years. The new document explicitly describes expectations that trainees will attain specific competencies as medical experts, in a range of levels:

- *Introductory knowledge* (ability to recognize identify or describe principles);
- *Working knowledge* (ability to demonstrate core aspects of psychiatry and understand the scientific literature);
- *Proficiency* (ability to demonstrate working knowledge enhanced by developmental cultural and lifespan perspective, allowing detailed interviewing and biopsychosocial problem formulation with capacity to teach, consult, assess and manage referrals as well as review the scientific literature).

These levels can be attained within the minimum training requirements. However, for levels beyond this, further training is required.

Advanced   Able to demonstrate detailed and sophisticated understanding, which is multimodal and interdisciplinary, leading to advanced

	teaching and consultation on complex referrals. Furthermore, the resident is able to apply and demonstrate familiarity and apply the scientific literature. It is felt that this level may be pursued as part of the selective and elective time.
Expert or master	Would require advanced training beyond core residency. This level is defined as leading to enhanced skills that enable management of patients with complex comorbidity treatment resistance or rare conditions. It is felt that the expert psychiatrist will have the capacity to review the literature critically, with enhanced expertise and generation of new questions for study.

The OTR, as with all other Royal College documents, reflects competencies in each of the seven CanMEDS roles.

The Specialty Training Requirements (STR) document for psychiatry, to be read in conjunction with the OTR, reflects many of the time-based changes made to the curriculum in the past few years. In this document, the full 60 months of approved residency training are tightly defined. The first (PGY I) or basic clinical training year (RCPSC, 2009b) emphasizes a broad-based medical experience relevant to psychiatry, with particular emphasis on experiences in internal medicine, family medicine, neurology and emergency medicine, as well as psychiatry.

The curriculum is to be considered as having junior residency (PGY II and PGY III year) and senior residency (PGY IV and PGY V) components, with a clear developmental trajectory of increasing maturity and competence as a psychiatrist.

The junior residency comprises basic and foundational training, with a focus on lifespan psychiatry in a variety of settings. This consists of twelve months of general psychiatry (inpatient and outpatient), six months of child psychiatry and six months of geriatric psychiatry (this latter increased from the previously mandated three months).

The senior residency (PGY IV and PGY V) involves the consolidation of core fundamental knowledge and skills, the assumption of more leadership and responsibility in supervision and education of junior colleagues, and an opportunity to develop career track interests through six months of elective and six months of selective training. Mandated experiences in the senior residency include three months of consultation and liaison psychiatry, the equivalent of two months of collaborative or shared care (family physicians and other professionals), and three to six months experience in treating patients with severe and persistent mental illness, including rehabilitation.

In addition, there are mandated longitudinal or horizontal requirements, including specific requirements in psychotherapy training (Weerasekera and Hnatko, 2009), addiction psychiatry and long-term follow-up of patients with severe and persistent mental illness.

The entire curriculum is to be taught and evaluated using the CanMEDS framework.

Table 10.1 Essential roles and key competencies of specialist physicians

Roles	Key competencies The specialist must be able to...
Medical expert	• Demonstrate diagnostic and therapeutic skills for ethical and effective patient care • Access and apply relevant information to clinical practice • Demonstrate effective consultation services with respect to patient care, education and legal opinions
Communicator	• Establish therapeutic relationship with patients, families • Obtain and synthesize relevant history from patients/families/communities • Listen effectively • Discuss appropriate information with patients/families and the healthcare team
Collaborator	• Consult effectively with other physicians and healthcare professionals • Contribute effectively to other interdisciplinary team activities
Manager	• Utilize resources effectively to balance patient care, learning needs, and outside activities • Allocate finite healthcare resources wisely • Work effectively and efficiently in a healthcare organization • Utilize information technology to optimize patient care, life-long learning and other activities
Health Advocate	• Identify the important determinants of health affecting patients • Contribute effectively to improved health of patients and communities • Recognize and respond to those issues where advocacy is appropriate
Scholar	• Develop, implement and monitor a personal continuing education strategy • Critically appraise sources of medical information • Facilitate learning of patients, house staff, students and other health professionals • Contribute to development of new knowledge
Professional	• Deliver highest quality care with integrity, honesty and compassion • Exhibit appropriate personal and interpersonal professional behaviours • Practise medicine ethically consistent with obligations of a physician

(Frank *et al.*, 1996)

Evaluation

Evaluation of each component of training occurs at mid-rotation and at the end of rotation. Block rotations are evaluated by means of an interim training evaluation report (ITER). Most programmes use an online version, which is printed off and forms part of the resident's file. Supervisors use a variety of methods to evaluate residents on rotation. These include but are not limited to direct observation, oral examinations (long case studies), OSCE, written examinations and multi-source feedback or 360-degree evaluation. This last method involves soliciting input from a variety of sources including multi-disciplinary staff, colleagues, peers and learners.

Most academic departments of psychiatry offer at least an annual formal evaluation day for residents, referred to as 'mock oral examination day', in which residents are examined using the diagnostic interview format and score sheet (RCPSC, 2006) (Appendix 10.1).

In addition, the standard for psychiatry residency programmes is to offer at least one and preferably two OSCEs per year. All residency programmes offer written examinations via the COPE exam, a national Canadian multiple-choice examination, and most programmes also offer the PRITE, a standardized North American multiple-choice examination. Residents receive written feedback on their performance on these examinations.

Other methods of evaluation have been developed to assess several of the Can-MEDS roles. Examples of these are the use of a CanMEDS portfolio, CanMEDS logs or tracking forms, projects (e.g., CQI projects as part of the 'manager' role), and preparation of a manuscript for publication or presentation at rounds of a scholarly review ('scholar' role). An example of a tracking form is the one used by McMaster University, for residents during their on-call night, in which they track numerous opportunities to fulfil and reflect on roles, such as 'health advocate' and 'manager' (Saperson and Brasch, private communication, 2007) (Appendix 10.2).

The evaluation methods used in the development of psychotherapeutic skills are comprehensively covered elsewhere in this book (see Chapter 11).

Changes to the final Royal College Examination in Psychiatry

Until 2001, the Royal College final examination in psychiatry that occurs at the end of the fifth year of residency consisted of a two-part examination. These were a written examination in the autumn and an oral examination offered twice a year in the final year of residency. The written examination was composed of two parts; approximately 175 multiple-choice questions and approximately ten short-answer questions. A pass in the written examination was required in order to sit the oral examination. The oral examination consisted of a two-hour diagnostic interview and discussion (The Royal College long case assessment). The format comprised a live interview with a patient of up to 55 minutes with one of the two examiners present in the interview room and the second observing by way of a two-way mirror. This was followed by a one-hour session, in which the candidate was required to present a summary of the history and mental status of the patient, as discovered in the examination, a case formulation, a differential diagnosis and a management plan. During this second hour, candidates were subject to questioning from two examiners. In earlier years, non-standardized case vignettes were an additional component.

In 2002, in keeping with educational standards aimed at greater reliability and validity, the examination format changed significantly. The premise for the change was the need for several sampling points. In addition, the RCPS decided to discontinue the involvement of live patients in final certification examinations in all specialties. The new format consisted of a single condensed examination, including both written and oral components. The written component continued to have both multiple-choice questions and short-answer questions. Success in this portion of the examination was no longer necessary for entrance to the oral examination section. The single long case examination was replaced by a number of stations or clinical encounters. These were initially referred to as PDM stations (phenomenology, diagnosis and management) but more recently the name was changed to 'OSCE' stations (objective structured clinical encounters). The current examination comprises approximately ten stations, each of which lasts approximately 20 minutes. An examiner is present in each station. The OSCE stations are used to assess:

Skills, knowledge and competence in a number of areas, including recognition of phenomenology, diagnostic skills, development of management plans, interpretation of laboratory radiological studies, the writing of consultation letters or reports, prescribing a treatment, oral presentation and communication skills, physical examination skills, psychotherapeutic skills and management skills. (RCPSC, 2007b)

The format of each station is variable and may include videotapes, laboratory investigation interpretations, written clinical vignettes followed by questions, role playing, and the creation of a consultation note or set of orders.

While the decision was made to remove the long case assessment from the final examination and replace it with several stations as a means of improving on reliability and validity, programme directors across the country were loth to allow it to disappear as an assessment method. They felt strongly that the long case assessment had significant face validity, and the skill set involved in the diagnostic interview was greatly valued by the profession, and so needed to be preserved. At the bi-annual meeting of the Programme Directors in Psychiatry (COPE, Coordinators of Psychiatric Education), programme directors from the 16 programmes across the country made a strong recommendation to the RCPS Specialty Committee in psychiatry to maintain the formal examination of the skill set involved in the diagnostic interview. This resulted in the development of a STACER (standard assessment of a clinical encounter report) in psychiatry, in which the long case examination became the responsibility of the programmes. Despite the fact that it was no longer a component of the final examination, residents were required to pass two long case diagnostic interviews (two out of a group of three orals, with a maximum of six attempts), in their final year of training, as part of the requirement for eligibility to sit the final examination.

There are ongoing challenges with administration of the STACER. The method of delivering and administering STACER examinations varies widely across the country. Residents have expressed concern at the perceived differences in standards across different programmes. At the bi-annual COPE meetings, the issue of the STACER continues to be vociferously debated, with proponents for and against a high-stake examination at the end of training. While there is overwhelming unanimous support for the preservation of the skill set involved in the long case assessment, current thinking among educators is leaning towards a 'stage-of-training'-specific oral examination, administered during the junior residency (PGY II and PGY III years) and again during the senior residency (PGY IV and PGY V years), for which specific developmental competencies can be defined and evaluated appropriate to the stage of training.

Residency training for international medical graduates

International medical graduates (IMGs) comprise approximately 20–30% of the physician workforce in Canada (Audas *et al.*, 2005). In Ontario, approximately 20% of the physician workforce consists of fully licensed international medical graduates. The Canadian task force on licensure of IMGs considered it important to include programmes of orientation to the cultural, legal and ethical organization of medicine in Canada and cultural and professional communication as elements in the preparation of IMGs for licensure. With a physician shortage in recent times, as well as Canada's historical reliance on IMGs, the task force regarded programmes that assist in preparing these physicians for the Canadian healthcare system to be an integral contribution to meeting Canadian healthcare needs (Monteiro *et al.*, private communication).

Most provinces in Canada have developed criteria and processes for screening international medical graduate applicants for residency programmes. In Ontario, all five residency programmes accept international medical graduates into the residency programme at varying levels. These include the first postgraduate year, entry at the second, third or fourth year of residency, and the 'practice-ready' level of entry. In the last level, IMGs undergo a six-month assessment in a recognized training programme prior to acceptance to sit the final Royal College Examination in Psychiatry and then enter into practice.

In the province of Ontario, the Centre for the Evaluation of Health Professionals Educated Abroad (CEHPEA), formerly known as IMG Ontario, was launched in 2007. The CEHPEA provides evaluation and orientation services to IMGs. These include pre-residency programmes for specialty residents, including psychiatry. The CEHPEA works in close collaboration with key stakeholders including the College of Physicians and Surgeons of Ontario (CPSO), the Royal College of Physicians and Surgeons of Canada (RCPSC), International Medical Graduate representatives, the Council of Ontario Faculties of Medicine (COFM) and other regulatory bodies of the various health professions. The CEHPEA also works in partnership with HealthForceOntario to help meet the demand for physicians (http://www.cehpea.ca).

International medical graduate residents are a heterogeneous group of learners, having diverse training experiences from a large number of countries. A growing number of IMGs are Canadian-born but have trained abroad. Given the heterogeneity of language and other socio-cultural factors, there are significant challenges in designing training and evaluation programmes to meet the needs of such a varied group.

Despite the pivotal role played by IMGs in the healthcare system, little is known about the issues that have an impact on their education and practice, and hence there are limited strategies and curricula available to help them address such issues (Rao *et al.*, 2007). In particular, there is limited understanding of the issues that IMGs face in the context of the Canadian healthcare culture, and limited research on the strategies that might be helpful to them in navigating the cultural and social hierarchical process and structural differences they may encounter (Monteiro *et al.*, private communication).

In response to the restricted amount of literature identifying evidence for effective curricula addressing acculturation communication skills, and the specific learning needs of IMG residents into the Canadian healthcare system, McMaster University's Department of Psychiatry and Behavioural Neurosciences has developed a proposed structured curriculum in psychiatry (Monteiro *et al.*, private communication). The curriculum has been developed to be delivered in three phases using qualitative and quantitative methodologies to evaluate the needs of IMGs and the effectiveness of the curriculum in meeting these needs. The curriculum is being implemented within a research protocol, providing IMGs the opportunity to discuss their own experiences of communicating in Canada as well as providing feedback on the content and process of the curriculum with suggestions for modification.

The curriculum is didactic and interactive, allowing IMGs to learn, practise and provide feedback on a variety of communication skills simultaneously. The proposed curriculum has five modules: the first module focuses on Canadian culture and strategies to address discrimination and Canadian healthcare culture; the second module addresses colloquialisms, metaphors and slang commonly heard in healthcare settings, strategies to overcome accent difficulties, small talk and empathic communication skills; the third module focuses on non-verbal behaviour appropriate in a Canadian healthcare context; the fourth module focuses on social and professional hierarchies in Canada and differences in communication between the opposite sexes; and the fifth module focuses on professional communications and includes such topics as ethics in medicine, boundary issues, privacy and confidentiality, dual relationships and feedback. The research component will have a mixed quantitative–qualitative methodology. The following tools will be used in addition to self-report satisfaction questionnaires:

1. **Acculturation** The Vancouver Index of Acculturation (Ryder *et al.*, 2000). This predicts psychosocial adjustment to Canada.
2. **Cross-cultural effectiveness** The Cross-Cultural Adaptability Scale (Kelley and Meyer, 1995) measures effectiveness in adjustment to a multicultural or cross-cultural setting.
3. **Observed communication behaviours** The Canadian Observed Communication Skills Scale (Appendix 10.3) consists of items generated from the empirical

literature on the assessment of empathy and communication skills, as well as North American and Canadian verbal and non-verbal communication norms. It is predicted that this measure will demonstrate changes in observed communication skills after the curriculum is administered.

It is hypothesized that this curriculum will provide evidence of efficacy in ensuring that IMG residents in psychiatry can successfully bridge the gaps identified between Canadian and internationally trained residents, and that IMGs are equipped to demonstrate comparable levels of competency in the final certification examination

Effective medical education, in keeping with universal trends of greater accountability, must adhere to standards of best practice and to the principles of best available evidence. Continuous evaluation of teaching methodologies, the increasing use of innovative and creative medical education techniques, flexible curricula and increasingly rigorous standards of accreditation are likely to continue to shape the future of psychiatric training. Collaborative and thoughtful sharing of resources from different systems of medical education will serve to enhance the quality of training available to psychiatry residents, to stimulate interest and recruit from among the best and the brightest of medical students, to destigmatize mental illness and, ultimately, to better serve our patients.

APPENDIX 10.1 RCPSC ORAL EXAMINATION SCORE SHEET FOR PSYCHIATRY

The Royal College of Physicians and Surgeons of Canada
Le Collège royal des médecins et chirurgiens du Canada
774 promenade Echo Drive, Ottawa, Canada K1S 5N8
Tel: (613) 730-8191 ✧ 1-800-668-3740 ✧ Fax: (613) 730-3707

RCPSC ORAL EXAMINATION SCORE SHEET FOR PSYCHIATRY

Date: _____   Time: _____
Candidates: _____
Examiner: _____

The oral examination tests the ability of the candidate to skillfully and compassionately address information that is needed to understand the patient in the context of his or her history and to establish a meaningful diagnosis and treatment plan, to synthesize the information obtained and to communicate this understanding:

(1)   **INTERVIEW PROCESS**   (to skillfully and compassionately address information)

Item	Unsatisfactory	B	Satisfactory
RAPPORT			
Establishes Relationship	Does not introduce self or exam. Uncertain. Does not assume control OR Begins asking closed questions.		Introduces self, explains interview. Begins in open, exploratory manner, Treats patient like a responsible adult.
Maintain professional therapeutic relationship	Mechanistic, distant, unresponsive disrespectful, patronizing.		Respectful. Genuinely interested. Eye contact, body posture suggests active listening.
INTERVIEW TECHNIQUE			
Information Gathering	Excessive closed or vague questions, Multiple simultaneous questions. Excessive jargon. Does not get detail. Uncomfortable with psychotic or sensitive material.		Mixes open and closed questions. Few leading or stacked questions. Asks clear questions in plain language.
Clarifies, follows up, confronts	Fails to try to clarify details of events, time sequences. Reluctant to challenge patient. Unsupportive when confronting patient.		Systematically tries to clarify details, unusual replies, inconsistencies. Pursues detail. Confronts inconsistencies supportively.
Attention/Listening	Talks over patient, OR passive, unsure leaving awkward silences. Does not make use of nonverbal material.		Practices receptive listening: allows silences and seems comfortable doing so.

The Royal College of Physicians and Surgeons of Canada
Le Collège royal des médecins et chirurgiens du Canada
774   promenade Echo Drive, Ottawa, Canada K1S 5N8
Tel: (613) 730-8191 ✧ 1-800-668-3740 ✧ Fax: (613) 730-3707

Item	Unsatisfactory	B	Satisfactory
Empathy	Fail to acknowledge patient distress, OR colludes or over-identifies with patient. Does not make use of non-verbal material.		Acknowledge distress with non-judgmental, empathic responses. Notes and responds to non-verbal cues.
Assuredness	Uncomfortable with feeling or psychotic content. Becomes flustered, freezes, or stifles such content.		At ease with affective, anxious or psychotic content of interview. Normalizes or helps patient understand symptoms.
Feedback, Interaction	Provides no feedback to patient, OR talks, educates, hypothesizes excessively.		Reframes, paraphrases. Summarizes understanding of story periodically. Gives a brief closing summary statement to patient.
ORGANIZATION			
Conducts orderly assessment / control	Inflexible, ignores patient needs, OR conducts a disorganized, disjointed interview. Allows patient to lead interview, drift, unable to focus.		Conducts structured but flexible interview, completing sections of interview in an orderly manner. Is able to politely redirect patient back to area under review, help patient focus.
Conducts comprehensive interview	Interview is not balanced. Focuses solely on principle problem, does not review for co-morbidity. Ignores the person in pursuit of symptoms. Fails to allocate time efficiently.		Conducts balanced interview. Gets clear sense of the person. Allocates time efficiently.

Rate the extent to which the candidate demonstrates interpersonal and interviewing skills at the level of a competent consultant general psychiatrist.

(at high end: 7 or more) Candidates engages well with the patient, facilitates communications with a good mix of open ended and specific questions, and responds adequately to verbal and non-verbal, especially affective cues: is receptive to important information that patient want to talk about, and asks about important things the patient does not volunteer but is not averse to talking about. Meets expectations. Errors or omissions are not major. A candidate around 9 or 10 does this, and helps patient overcome obstacles.

(at low end: 6 or less) Candidate fails to engage well with the patient, and does not facilitate communication or interferes with what patient want to say. For example, uses excessive structure (e.g. closed ended or multiple choice questions, or does not respond adequately to verbal or non-verbal, especially affective cues).

0 ____ 1 ____ 2 ____ 3 ____ 4 ____ 5 ____ 6 ____ 7 ____ 8 ____ 9 ____ 10 ____

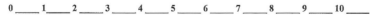

The Royal College of Physicians and Surgeons of Canada
Le Collège royal des médecins et chirurgiens du Canada
774 promenade Echo Drive, Ottawa, Canada K1S 5N8
Tel: (613) 730-8191 ✧ 1-800-668-3740 ✧ Fax: (613) 730-3707

(2)   **INTERVIEW CONTENT** (information that is needed...)

Item	Unsatisfactory	B	Satisfactory
HPI Premorbid state	Fails to address pre-morbid state		Adequately addresses pre-morbid state
Illness Onset	Fails to address circumstances of onset of illness / episode		Addresses stressors and time of onset of illness
Symptoms and Course of Episode	Does not adequately attempt to identify symptoms or clarify evolution of current illness.		Addresses symptoms of current episode / illness, and does not blur this with previous episodes.
			For a stable patient with no current episode, assesses current level of symptoms and functioning.
Therapeutic Interventions	Fails to address therapeutic interventions		Addresses therapeutic interventions in current episode
Comorbidity Screening	Preoccupied with a single diagnosis. Does not screen for comorbidity		Reviews criteria for symptoms of likely differential diagnoses and likely comorbid diagnoses.
SAFETY	Fails to assess or minimizes risk of self-harm, aggression or self care OR exaggerates seriousness of threat.		Asks about suicidality, aggressivity, competency to care for self, IF indicated by patient's mental status during interview.
Risk Assessment	Fails to review risk factors, OR reviews in depth when not warranted.		Systematically reviews risk factors for suicide, self-harm, self-care, harm to others, IF INDICATED. Does not do so if not required.
MEDS	Does not ask about medication		Asks about current medications: dose, duration, effectiveness, side effects.
PSYCH-HISTORY			
Past Episodes	Fails to review		Reviews previous episodes, hospitalizations, evolution of illness, aggression and self-harm.
Treatments	Fails to review		Reviews past treatments, including therapists and relationship to them: medications including dose, duration, efficacy, side effects, and compliance; other treatments.
Substance Use	Fails to review		Reviews substance use-abuse
Forensic History	Fails to review		Reviews legal involvements, if indicated
FAMILY PSYCH HISTORY	Fails to review		Reviews family psychiatric history including substance abuse
MEDICAL HISTORY	Fails to review		Reviews medical history, including allergies, serious drug reactions in past, response to illness

The Royal College of Physicians and Surgeons of Canada
Le Collège royal des médecins et chirurgiens du Canada
774   promenade Echo Drive, Ottawa, Canada K1S 5N8
Tel: (613) 730-8191 ✧ 1-800-668-3740 ✧ Fax: (613) 730-3707

Item	Unsatisfactory	B	Satisfactory
GROWTH, PERSONAL HX	Fails to review		Reviews only childhood and adolescent development and relationships, including abuse
	Fails to review		Reviews academic achievement and work history, and current functioning
	Fails to review		Reviews adult relationships, including current relationship and supports
MSE	Omits important areas, or performs mental status exam when not indicated		Conducts formal mental status exam if indicated. Does not do so if not indicated. Cover relevant content areas.

Rate the extent to which the relevant content areas have been addresses at the level of a competent consultant general psychiatrist.

(at high end: 7 or more) Candidate addresses most important areas needed for understanding the patient's illness in context, and arriving at multidimensional treatment plan. These are addressed with reasonable balance, in sufficient depth and in an organized manner. Omissions are not critical. (9 or 10): Most areas thoroughly and competently addresses.

(at low end: 6 or less) Candidate omits important areas, or addresses important area in insufficient depth. Interview lacks adequate structure or organization.

0 _____ 1 _____ 2 _____ 3 _____ 4 _____ 5 _____ 6 _____ 7 _____ 8 _____ 9 _____ 10 _____

(3)   **UNDERSTANDING**   (...ability...to synthesize the information obtained to
understand the patient in the context of his/her history, to establish a meaningful diagnosis and
management plan...)

Unsatisfactory	B	Satisfactory
DIAGNOSIS		
Proposes a diagnosis or principle problem unsupported by the interview		Provides a realistic diagnosis supported by evidence from the interview.
Unable to present or defend a differential diagnosis, OR provides an overinclusive differential, stressing the esoteric		Provides a brief and realistic differential diagnosis and is able to explain process of further clarifying the diagnosis.
Is inflexible in discussing diagnoses. Is unable to entertain alternatives.		Able to discuss difficulties in supporting and refuting diagnoses in a thoughtful, balanced manner.
Is unaware of issues related to comorbidity		Is able to discuss comorbidity and interplay between diagnoses.
Unsatisfactory	B	Satisfactory

The Royal College of Physicians and Surgeons of Canada
Le Collège royal des médecins et chirurgiens du Canada
774   promenade Echo Drive, Ottawa, Canada K1S 5N8
Tel: (613) 730-8191 ✧ 1-800-668-3740 ✧ Fax: (613) 730-3707

FORMULATION		
Is unable to provide a summative understanding of the patient. Focuses narrowly on a single aspect of phase of the illness.		Identifies predisposing, precipitating, perpetuating factors for patient's problem, described in a manner which recreates a while person and his/her life.
View of patient neglects key components of his/her life, is unduly limited in its grasp. Uninterested in patient as an individual person		Able to identify biopsychosocial components of patient's illness, and describe the interplay between these elements at this time.
Is unable to identify dynamic or cognitive factors influencing patient's presentation		Able to identify come conflicts, cognitive distortions, dependency of interpersonal needs of the patient.
MANAGEMENT		
Treatment plan has no clear goals or expected outcomes. Plan is unrealistic for the patient, or is not attainable in existing mental health system		Provides realistic treatment plan covering short term, medium term and long term goals of treatment
Has very limited understanding of indications for and limitations of pharmacotherapy and other biological therapies. Recommends inappropriate biological treatments without understanding of risks and benefits. Lacks evidence for efficacy of treatment proposed.		Able to recommend and defend SPECIFIC pharmacotherapies, if indicated. Aware of evidence for efficacy of therapy provided.
Unaware of indications for and limitations of specific types of psychotherapy. Recommends inappropriate therapy.		Able to recommend and defend prescription of SPECIFIC psychotherapies, if relevant.
Has poor understanding of long term prospects for patient. Provides unrealistic outcomes, little understanding of real life, day to day management issues.		Able to provide realistic prognosis. Able to describe barriers to compliance / effective intervention with THIS patient.

Rate the extent to which the candidate demonstrates competence in understanding, diagnosing, and managing this patient at the level of a competent consultant general psychiatrist.

(at high end: 7 or more) Candidate shows good understanding of patient's illness in the context of patient's life. Conclusions are based on evidence. Candidate addresses biological, psychological, and social aspects of management in knowledgeable, relevant manner. (Any Bs and Us are not major).

(at low end: 6 or less) Candidate's answers are imprecise or formulaic. Does not take into account the particular individual patient.

0 _____ 1 ____ 2 ____ 3 ____ 4 ____ 5 ____ 6 ____ 7 ____ 8 ____ 9 ____ 10 ____

The Royal College of Physicians and Surgeons of Canada
Le Collège royal des médecins et chirurgiens du Canada
774 promenade Echo Drive, Ottawa, Canada K1S 5N8
Tel: (613) 730-8191 ✧ 1-800-668-3740 ✧ Fax: (613) 730-3707

(4)   **PRESENTATION**   (ability to communicate this understanding...)

Unsatisfactory	B	Satisfactory
Case is disorganized or a simple repetition of symptoms without a unifying story line or sense of the person. Time sequences mix current with past episodes.		Case is presented in an orderly, systematic manner. Presentation successfully tells the patient's story. Paints a clear picture of the course of illness.
Symptoms are not clustered to aid with diagnosis, OR symptoms are presented in excessive detail.		Presentation includes relevant positive and negative symptoms needed to support the diagnosis.
Case is rambling and overinclusive, OR presentation is unduly brief and uninformative.		Case presentation is concise, but includes relevant detail and texture.
Rigid, inflexible, confrontational in discussion. Unable to entertain other possibilities OR unable to take a position for discussion. Immediately accepts examiner's viewpoint.		Demonstrates capacity for open-mindedness, thoughtful discussion of issues identified.

Rate the candidate's presentation and discussion at the level of a competent consultant general psychiatrist.

(at high end: 7 or more) Presentation is organized, focused and relevant. Answers are precise and relate to the patient seen.

(at lower end: 6 or less) Presentation is disorganized or overinclusive. Vague.

0 _____ 1_____ 2 _____ 3 _____ 4 _____ 5 _____ 6 _____ 7 _____ 8 _____ 9 _____ 10 _____

Errors of Omission or Commission that would

1)   endanger the patient or others
2)   seriously compromise the relationship with the patient
3)   lead to an incorrect of inadequate assessment of the patient's problem (e.g. missing a
       major abnormality on history or examination)

If yes, please comment:

_____
_____
_____
_____

Overall

Rate this candidate's performance at the level of the consultant general psychiatrist

Meets expectations _____   B _____   Below expectations _____
                          .70   65 - 69   <65

The Royal College of Physicians and Surgeons of Canada
Le Collège royal des médecins et chirurgiens du Canada
774   promenade Echo Drive, Ottawa, Canada K1S 5N8
Tel: (613) 730-8191 ✧ 1-800-668-3740 ✧ Fax: (613) 730-3707

OVERALL PERFORMANCE
IN-TRAINING COMPREHENSIVE PSYCHIATRIC ASSESSMENT

Name: _____   University: _____

This resident has successfully completed two comprehensive psychiatric assessments, as described in the Guidelines and scored using the RCPSC Oral Examination Score Sheet for Psychiatry, during the last twelve months. The completed score sheets are to be retained by the program as part of the resident's evaluation record.

The following is a summary, compiled by the program director, of the performance on these assessments with comments on strengths and weaknesses.

Strengths:

_____
_____
_____
_____
_____

Weaknesses:

_____
_____
_____
_____
_____

_____   _____
(Print) Name of Program Director   Date

_____   _____
Signature of Program Director   Resident's Signature

THIS DOCUMENT IS TO BE RETURNED WITH THE FITER.

APPENDIX 10.2 CANMEDS COMPETENCIES SELF-REFLECTIVE JOURNAL

CanMEDS Competencies Self-Reflective Journal

Date on call: _____ Senior Resident:_____
    Junior Resident: _____
Clinical Clerks: _____
Clinicians/nurses: _____
On-Call Adult Psychiatrist: _____ Attended in person : Yes __ No __Time_____
On-Call Child Psychiatrist _____   Attended in person : Yes __ No __Time_____

CanMeds roles practiced while on call.

☐ **Medical Expert**	☐ **Communicator**	☐ **Scholar**
Collaborator ☐ Shared decision making ☐ Shared knowledge & Information ☐Delegation ☐ Respect for other team members ☐ Constructive negotiation ☐ Leadership based on patient needs ☐ Conflict resolution, management or prevention ☐ Collaborate with ER ☐ Collaborate with community agency ☐ Learning together ☐ Other _____	**Manager** ☐ Supervision of team members ☐ Triage ☐ Effective time management ☐ Negotiation ☐ Allocate scarce resources (eg inpatient beds) ☐ Other _____	
Health Advocate ☐ Health promotion ☐ Fiduciary duty to care ☐ Mobilize resources ☐ Patient safety ☐ Determinants of health ☐ Advocacy for patient(s) ☐ Other _____	**Professional** ☐Altruism ☐ Integrity & honesty ☐ Compassion & caring ☐ Self-awareness ☐ Disclosure of error or adverse event ☐ Ethical issues ☐ Patient confidentiality issues ☐ Boundary issues ☐ Other_____	

Reflect on one CanMeds role practiced on call

© Psychiatry McMaster University

APPENDIX 10.3 THE CANADIAN OBSERVED COMMUNICATION SKILLS SCALE

MEASURE TO RATE CANADIAN COMMUNICATION SKILLS IN THE CLINICAL ENCOUNTERS OF INTERNATIONAL MEDICAL GRADUATE STUDENTS IN CANADIAN SETTINGS

(Independent Rater Measure)

I am (Please circle one):   Rater 1   Rater 2

Student Number:

Instructions:

On the following pages there are sentences that describe some of the different communication skills health professional use in an encounter with a client. After you watch a health professional engage a simulated patient, please evaluate the person on the following communication skills.

Below each statement inside there is a seven point scale:

1	2	3	4	5	6	7
Never	Rarely	Occasionally	Sometimes	Often	Very Often	Always

Please circle the number that best represents your evaluation of the person's ability on that communication skill.

The information in this questionnaire is CONFIDENTIAL and should not be given to the professional or the simulated patient. Please complete all the items on this questionnaire. Place the questionnaire in an envelope and return it to Dr. Althea Monteiro.

Verbal Behavior:

1. The professional addressed the patient appropriately (for example, asked if they could use their first name, used first name if the person was young or around the same age, or used Mr./Ms. if the person was older).

1	2	3	4	5	6	7
Never	Rarely	Occasionally	Sometimes	Often	Very Often	Always

2. The professional introduced themselves including their profession.

1	2	3	4	5	6	7
Never	Rarely	Occasionally	Sometimes	Often	Very Often	Always

3. The professional was polite (for example, apologized if they were late or interrupted, said please, thank you, and goodbye).

1	2	3	4	5	6	7
Never	Rarely	Occasionally	Sometimes	Often	Very Often	Always

4. The professional engaged the patient appropriately from the beginning to the end of the interview.

1	2	3	4	5	6	7
Never	Rarely	Occasionally	Sometimes	Often	Very Often	Always

5. The professional negotiated and clarified the purpose of the meeting and the patient's goals.

1	2	3	4	5	6	7
Never	Rarely	Occasionally	Sometimes	Often	Very Often	Always

6. The professional explicitly structured the meeting with the patient as appropriate.

1	2	3	4	5	6	7
Never	Rarely	Occasionally	Sometimes	Often	Very Often	Always

7. The professional questioned the patient appropriately (i.e. asked direct and concrete questions, and moved from open-ended to close-ended questions).

1	2	3	4	5	6	7
Never	Rarely	Occasionally	Sometimes	Often	Very Often	Always

8. The professional communicated in a clear and concise manner (e.g., explained any jargon used or avoided jargon in the first place).

1	2	3	4	5	6	7
Never	Rarely	Occasionally	Sometimes	Often	Very Often	Always

8.

9. The professional encouraged the patient to ask questions and express his/her feelings.

1	2	3	4	5	6	7
Never	Rarely	Occasionally	Sometimes	Often	Very Often	Always

10. The professional summarized information for patient.

1	2	3	4	5	6	7
Never	Rarely	Occasionally	Sometimes	Often	Very Often	Always

11. The professional used silence effectively to facilitate patient communication.

1	2	3	4	5	6	7
Never	Rarely	Occasionally	Sometimes	Often	Very Often	Always

12. The professional used transitional statements to go from one topic to another.

1	2	3	4	5	6	7
Never	Rarely	Occasionally	Sometimes	Often	Very Often	Always

13. The professional used suggestive or persuasive statements rather than directive statements when appropriate.

1	2	3	4	5	6	7
Never	Rarely	Occasionally	Sometimes	Often	Very Often	Always

Vocal Qualities:

14. The professional spoke clearly (i.e. enunciated their words and spoke at a medium to slow rate).

1	2	3	4	5	6	7
Never	Rarely	Occasionally	Sometimes	Often	Very Often	Always

15. The professional ensured that the content of their message was congruent with vocal tone.

1	2	3	4	5	6	7
Never	Rarely	Occasionally	Sometimes	Often	Very Often	Always

16. The professional attempted to maintain a medium pitch in their voice and medium volume of voice most of the time.

1	2	3	4	5	6	7
Never	Rarely	Occasionally	Sometimes	Often	Very Often	Always

Body Position and Body Language

17. The professional kept their attention focused on the patient and their face turned towards the patient for most of the interview. (For example, they did not indicate boredom or disinterest, for example, through yawns or by engaging in other tasks while speaking with the patient).

1	2	3	4	5	6	7
Never	Rarely	Occasionally	Sometimes	Often	Very Often	Always

18. The professional used open, interested body language (For example, they leaned forward slightly, kept their arms by their side when not writing notes or conducting an examination, and did not cross their arms)

1	2	3	4	5	6	7
Never	Rarely	Occasionally	Sometimes	Often	Very Often	Always

19. The professional maintained a relaxed and upright body position and appropriate distance between his/herself and the patient (approximately 14 inches).

1	2	3	4	5	6	7
Never	Rarely	Occasionally	Sometimes	Often	Very Often	Always

20. The professional allowed their note taking to interfere with their dialogue with the patient.

1	2	3	4	5	6	7
Never	Rarely	Occasionally	Sometimes	Often	Very Often	Always

21. The professional engaged in inappropriate physical contact with the patient (for example, patting the patient's hand or back, holding their hand for more than a brief length of time, putting an arm around the patient, etc).

1	2	3	4	5	6	7
Never	Rarely	Occasionally	Sometimes	Often	Very Often	Always

22. The professional used appropriate verbal and non-verbal gestures (For example, smiling when appropriate, nodding in encouragement, looking concerned when appropriate).

1	2	3	4	5	6	7
Never	Rarely	Occasionally	Sometimes	Often	Very Often	Always

Empathic behavior

23. The professional made an effort to understand the patient's explanation of his/her difficulties (i.e. used statements such as "Am I understanding you correctly?")

1	2	3	4	5	6	7
Never	Rarely	Occasionally	Sometimes	Often	Very Often	Always

24. The professional conveyed warmth to the patient through his/her tone.

1	2	3	4	5	6	7
Never	Rarely	Occasionally	Sometimes	Often	Very Often	Always

25. The professional made an effort to ensure that the patient understood him/her (i.e. used questions of clarification)

1	2	3	4	5	6	7
Never	Rarely	Occasionally	Sometimes	Often	Very Often	Always

26. The professional conveyed genuineness in his/her responses to the patient.

1	2	3	4	5	6	7
Never	Rarely	Occasionally	Sometimes	Often	Very Often	Always

27. The professional listened attentively to the patient.

1	2	3	4	5	6	7
Never	Rarely	Occasionally	Sometimes	Often	Very Often	Always

28. The professional used mirroring appropriately (e.g., repeating key words used by patient, matching patient's voice tone and intensity).

1	2	3	4	5	6	7
Never	Rarely	Occasionally	Sometimes	Often	Very Often	Always

29. The professional communications included a number of assumptions he/she made about the client's difficulties.

1	2	3	4	5	6	7
Never	Rarely	Occasionally	Sometimes	Often	Very Often	Always

30. The professional maintained appropriate eye contact with the patient.

1	2	3	4	5	6	7
Never	Rarely	Occasionally	Sometimes	Often	Very Often	Always

31. The professional conveyed verbal and/or non-verbal disgust or distaste for the client information the client was discussing.

1	2	3	4	5	6	7
Never	Rarely	Occasionally	Sometimes	Often	Very Often	Always

REFERENCES

Audas, R., Ross, A. and Vardy, D. (2005). The use of provisionally licensed medical graduates in Canada. *Canadian Medical Association Journal*, **173**(11), 1315–1316.

Frank, J. R. (2005). *The CanMEDS 2005 Physician Competency Framework. Better Standards. Better Physicians. Better Care.* Ottawa: The Royal College of Physicians and Surgeons of Canada. http://rcpsc.medical.org./canmeds/CanMEDS2005/CanMEDS2005_e.pdf.

Frank, J. R., Jabbour, M., Tugwell, P. *et al.* (1996). *Skills for the New Millennium: Report of the Societal Needs Working Group, CanMEDS 2000 Project.* Ottawa: The Royal College of Physicians and Surgeons of Canada. http://rcpsc.medical.org/canmeds/CanMEDS_e. pdf.

Kelley, C. and Meyer, J. (1995). *CCAI Manual: Cross-Cultural Adaptability Inventory.* Arlington VA,: Vangent Inc.

Leverette, J. S. (2009). The road to renewal in postgraduate education in psychiatry. In *Approaches to Postgraduate Education in Psychiatry in Canada*, ed. J. S. Leverette, G. S. Hnatko and E. Persad, 1st edn. Ottawa: Canadian Psychiatric Association, pp. 1–14.

Rae-Grant, Q. (ed.) (1996). *Images in Psychiatry: Canada.* Washington: American Psychiatric Association.

Rao, N. R., Kramer, M., Saunders, R. *et al.* (2007). An annotated bibliography of professional literature on international medical graduates. *Academic Psychiatry*, **31**(1), 68–83.

RCPSC (Royal College of Physicians and Surgeons of Canada) (2006). *RCPSC Oral Examination Score Sheet for Psychiatry.* http://rcpsc.medical.org/residency/certification/ stacers/psychiatry_e.pdf.

RCPSC (Royal College of Physicians and Surgeons of Canada) (2007a). *The CanMEDS Roles Framework Diagram.* http://rcpsc.medical.org/canmeds/index.php.

RCPSC (Royal College of Physicians and Surgeons of Canada) (2007b). *Format of the Comprehensive Objective Examination in Psychiatry.* http://rcpsc.medical.org/residency/ certification/examformats/165_e.php.

RCPSC (Royal College of Physicians and Surgeons of Canada) (2009a). *RCPS Education and Continuing Professional Development.* http://rcpsc.medical.org/residency/.

RCPSC (Royal College of Physicians and Surgeons of Canada) (2009b). *Specialty Training Requirements in Psychiatry.* Royal College of Physicians and Surgeons of Canada. http://rcpsc.medical.org/residency/certification/training/psychiatry_e.pdf.

Ryder, A. G., Alden, L. E. and Paulhaus, D. L. (2000). Is acculturation unidimensional or bidimensional? A head-to-head comparison is prediction of personality, self-identity, and adjustment. *Journal of Personality and Social Psychology*, **9**(1), 49–65.

Swinson, R. P. and Leverette, J. S. (2009). The evolution of training in general psychiatry and its relationship to subspecialization within psychiatry. In *Approaches to Postgraduate*

Education in Psychiatry in Canada, ed. J. S. Leverette, G. S. Hnatko and E. Persad. 1st edn. Ottawa: Canadian Psychiatric Association, pp. 15–33.

Weerasekera, P. and Hnatko, G. S. (2009). Psychotherapies. In *Approaches to Postgraduate Education in Psychiatry in Canada*, ed. J. S. Leverette, G. S. Hnatko and E. Persad. 1st edn. Ottawa: Canadian Psychiatric Association, pp. 71–88.

11

Workplace-based assessment in psychotherapy: a Canadian experience

Priyanthy Weerasekera

Editors' introduction

Assessment of psychotherapy skills are often neglected within postgraduate psychiatric programmes. This is mainly because of logistic and resource issues, as well as a lack of local expertise in assessing these complex skills. Here, Weerasekera describes in great detail the unique, excellent and evidence-based psychotherapy training and assessment programmes for psychiatric trainees at McMaster University in Canada. Some validated assessment tools that can be used in assessments of trainee performance in different psychotherapeutic techniques are also outlined here. Finally, the institutional support factors that have contributed to the success of the McMaster programme are also discussed.

Introduction

Psychotherapy is psychological treatment that benefits patients with psychiatric disorders. Meta-analyses and randomized control trials support the use of cognitive-behavioural therapies (CBT) in mood, anxiety, eating and psychotic disorders (Butler *et al.*, 2006; Cuijpers *et al.*, 2008), interpersonal therapy (IPT) for depression (de Mello *et al.*, 2005), psychodynamic therapy for a variety of disorders (Leichsenring and Rabung, 2008), dialectical behaviour therapy (DBT) for borderline personality disorder (BPD) (Binks *et al.*, 2006), motivational interviewing (MI) for substance abuse conditions (Hettema *et al.*, 2005), couple and family therapy as an adjunct for child and adult disorders (Shadish and Baldwin, 2003) and group therapies for mood, anxiety, eating and other disorders (Burlingame *et al.*, 2003).

As a result of these developments in the empirical literature and the Canadian emphasis on evidence-based medicine, significant revisions have been made to training requirements in psychotherapy. Current guidelines stipulate that residents must be exposed to the evidence-based psychotherapies with *proficiency* (prime therapist with supervision) in supportive, crisis intervention, CBT, psychodynamic and family or group therapy; *working knowledge* (co-therapist or observation) in behavioural, DBT, IPT, and family or group therapy; and *introductory knowledge* (no clinical exposure required) in brief dynamic, mindfulness, motivational interviewing and relaxation (RCPSC, 2007, p.7). Attention has also been given to empathy, rapport, trust and the development of ethical therapeutic relationships with patients. The objective in widening the training requirements is to train a more sophisticated general psychiatrist. Some assistance has been provided to help training directors meet these new guidelines (Weerasekera and Hnatko, 2009).

Similar changes have also occurred in the United States. The Accreditation Council on Graduate Medical Education (ACGME) recently mandated that all psychiatric residents must:

Develop competence in applying supportive, psychodynamic and CBT to both brief and long term individual practice, as well as to assuring exposure to family, couples, group and other individual evidence-based psychotherapies. (ACGME, 2007, p. 15)

In the United Kingdom, the Royal College of Psychiatrists clearly state that:

The doctor will also demonstrate the ability to conduct a range of individual, group and family therapies using standard accepted models and to integrate these psychotherapies into everyday treatment, including biological and socio-cultural interventions. (RCP, 2009)

They must also:

Demonstrate mastery of the theory, technique, and application of a recognized form of psychotherapy (CBT, psychodynamic or systemic) . . . as well as develop competence in the theory and technique of two other recognized forms of psychotherapy. (RCP, 2009, p. 16)

Therefore, UK residents must reach mastery level in one form of psychotherapy and competence in two others.

The shift in training requirements in psychotherapy has led to considerable discussion amongst educators in the field (Yager and Bienenfeld, 2003). Attention has been given to conceptual issues concerning the definition of therapies, and practical issues focusing on the assessment of competence (Bienenfeld *et al.*, 2003). For the psychotherapies, manuals have been developed to provide operational definitions readily available for clinical use. Assessing competence, however, is more challenging and controversial, and minimal guidelines have been provided.

In psychotherapy, *competence* is defined as the therapist's level of skill in delivering a particular treatment, whereas *adherence* refers to the extent that techniques employed in therapy match those described in a manual (Waltz *et al.*, 1993). Competence assumes adherence to specific techniques and a good working alliance. Importantly, rigid adherence to protocols is negatively related to competence in many therapies (Henry *et al.*, 1993). Competence in psychotherapy also implies a

good understanding of theory, the treatment outcome literature and the maintenance of professional behaviours. Defining an acceptable level of competence for a
trainee is challenging. Most residents should be able to attain beginning skills in a
variety of therapies with advanced skills in one or two therapies. It will be difficult,
however, for a trainee to perform at a master therapist level and this requires many
years of training and experience.

Historically in psychotherapy, resident competence has been assessed when the
resident and supervisor review session process notes together. This is not a valid
and reliable method of assessment, as process notes discussed in supervision tend
to accentuate positive aspects of therapy and minimize those that contribute to
ruptures in the alliance (Chevron et al., 1983). It is also difficult to provide specific feedback regarding therapeutic technique with this method of evaluation.
Assessment of competence should therefore be based on a variety of sources and
methods. Supervisors need to be presented with session material they can see or
at least hear, so that specific feedback can be given and competence assessed. An
'objective' evaluation is also essential, whereby an unbiased evaluator assesses performance based on clearly defined criteria for competence. These 'criteria' have
been established by competence rating scales which can be utilized in training
institutions, as long as modifications are made to fit expectations from residents.
These scales however, do not take into account such contextual variables as patient
characteristics, therapist characteristics, presenting problem and stage of therapy;
all important variables when assessing therapist competence. Despite these difficulties, these scales provide us with some objective means to assess specific skills,
and can be used in conjunction with other more qualitative evaluation methods
to assess overall competence in psychotherapy.

This chapter discusses an empirically oriented, broad-based, standardized, competency-focused psychotherapy training programme in Hamilton,
Canada. The basic principles of this programme have been described elsewhere
(Weerasekera et al., 2003), with preliminary data on resident competence presented
in an earlier publication (Weerasekera, 1997). This chapter will focus on the current programme, which has been revised to meet the current RCPSC guidelines. A
brief description of each modality and specific instruments used to assess competence will be presented. The advantages and disadvantages of such a programme
will also be discussed.

The McMaster psychotherapy programme

Table 11.1 outlines the original empirically oriented, competency-based psychotherapy training programme developed at McMaster University (Weerasekera,
1997). At the time, this programme represented a significant shift from the Royal
College guidelines, which emphasized training in long-term psychodynamic psychotherapy. Over time, programme modifications were made that reflected developments in the literature. Emotion-focused therapy (EFT) replaced client-centred

Table 11.1 McMaster psychotherapy programme, 1995

Year	Rotation	Sequence of module	Seminars	Therapist rating scale	Number of supervisors	Number of assessors
PGY-2	Inpatient or outpatient	Client-centred therapy	Client-centred therapy	Truax Accurate Empathy Rating Scale	2	2
	Inpatient or outpatient	CBT anxiety and depression	CBT	Cognitive therapy scale (CTS)	3	2
PGY-3	Child	Family	Family	Family therapy rating scale (FTRS)	4	2
	Chronic care	Psychodynamic	Psychodynamic		6	
PGY-4	Geriatrics	Interpersonal therapy (IPT)	IPT	Therapist strategy rating form (TSRF)	2	2
	Consultation	Couple	Couple		2	
PGY-5	Elective	Group	Group		4	

therapy, since the former not only taught alliance-building skills but showed superior outcomes in the treatment of depression (Ellison *et al.*, 2009), and dealt with specific depression-related issues (e.g., loss, unfinished business with a significant other or problematic reactions). Additional therapies were also added as electives, such as DBT, brief dynamic therapy and motivational interviewing. Many of these therapies are now compulsory, given the current RCPSC guidelines. And finally couple therapy was changed from a mandatory to an elective module.

Assessment of competence in psychotherapy

The McMaster University programme has always maintained a standardized approach to training with a heavy emphasis on the assessment of competence. With the exception of long-term psychodynamic therapy, all therapies are clearly defined and their implementation documented in appropriate manuals. All therapy sessions are audiotaped, or in some cases videotaped or screened live, and assessed weekly by the supervisor, who has been specifically trained in that module. Recorded material is played back during feedback sessions, permitting supervisors to give moment-to-moment feedback to the resident. Therefore, the assessment of competence is based on ongoing evaluation of segments of the resident's performance data, rather than solely on the resident's *impression* of the session. More importantly, for those therapies with established therapist rating scales, residents submit early and late session tapes for evaluation by an alternate supervisor, who blindly rates these tapes utilizing an empirically validated therapist competence rating scale. A minimum of two assessors per module is required for this purpose.

Given the expansion of the training requirements and the rigorous evaluation process, assessment of competence using therapist rating scales is carried out for one case per module. A resident who fails to meet the competency requirement of a module is required to repeat the module. Skills learned in the 'test case' are generalized to other cases throughout the resident's training, and for these cases competence is assessed only by the supervisor. Many residents carry several cases throughout their training in different placements, and have the opportunity to 'specialize' in one or two modules in the senior or fellowship year.

It is important to mention that the assessment of competence is not based solely on performance on therapist rating scales, but includes faculty evaluation of the resident's performance in supervision sessions and seminars. Using our own evaluation forms we assess a resident's general and specific psychotherapy skills, knowledge base and professional behaviours.

Faculty staff, comprising psychiatrists, psychologists and social workers, are also assessed for their supervisory and seminar presentation skills. Supervision is offered individually or in groups where resources are limited, the latter being favourably received by the residents, who enjoy learning with their colleagues. We have increased the complement of supervisors mostly through in-house training and recruitment. Residents have consistently rated supervision as very good or excellent and seminars as above average (Weerasekera *et al.*, 2003). It is significant that both supervision and seminar satisfaction ratings have improved over time. We would like to attribute this to the annual changes that are made as a result of our ongoing evaluation process and resident input.

Table 11.2 illustrates the current programme and outlines the sequence of training and the instruments used to assess competence. This programme meets the current RCPSC guidelines. Next is a discussion of how we assess relationship skills, as defined by the therapeutic alliance; empathic skills; and therapeutic skills specific to each form of psychotherapy.

Therapeutic alliance

The therapeutic alliance is defined as the fundamental relationship between the therapist and the patient, and is made up of three components: a bond (relational component), mutually agreed goals, and tasks (means to attain goals) (Bordin, 1979). Three decades of research demonstrate that a positive therapeutic alliance is essential for good outcomes in psychotherapy (Horvath, 2001). Research also shows that the alliance is essential for good outcomes in pharmacotherapy

Table 11.2 McMaster psychotherapy programme, 2009

Year	Rotation	Sequence of module	Seminars	Therapist rating scale	Number of supervisors	Number of assessors
BCT	ER	Crisis intervention	Crisis intervention		2	
PGY-2	Inpatient	Emotion-focused therapy (EFT)	EFT	Truax Accurate Empathy Scale	4	2
	Outpatient	CBT – depression CBT – anxiety	CBT depression and anxiety	Cognitive therapy scale (CTS)	8	2
PGY-3	Chronic	Psychodynamic	Psychodynamic	Psychodynamic rating scale	10	2
	Child	Family	Family	Family therapy rating scale (FTRS)	4	2
		Motivational interviewing	Motivational interviewing	Motivational interviewing skills code (MISC)	4	2
PGY-4	Geriatrics, consult	Interpersonal therapy (IPT)	IPT	Therapist strategy rating form (TSRF)	2	2
	Elective	Group (dialectical behavioural therapy)	Group (DBT and other)		7	
PGY-5	Elective	Electives	Integration			

(Weiss *et al.*, 2002). Therapist attributes (warmth, genuineness, respectfulness and being empathic) and techniques (empathic reflection, affective exploration, supportiveness, facilitation of the expression of affect and attention to the patient's experience) have an impact on a positive outcome in therapy and are specific skills that should be taught and assessed in training (Ackerman and Hilsenroth, 2003). Therapies that pay specific attention to these training variables include supportive (Winston *et al.*, 2004), client-centred (Rogers, 1965), emotion-focused (Greenberg *et al.*, 1993), supportive–expressive (Luborsky, 1984) and self-psychologically oriented psychodynamic therapy (Rowe and MacIsaac, 1991). Therapist competence in the alliance, and alliance-related skills (e.g., empathy) can be assessed by such instruments as the Working Alliance Inventory (WAI) (Horvath and Greenberg, 1994), the Barrett–Lennard Relationship Inventory (Simmons *et al.*, 1995) and the Truax Accurate Empathy Scale (Truax, 1976).

Over the past three years we have been using the Working Alliance Inventory in all individual psychotherapy modules. Patients are administered the WAI around the third session and again towards the end of treatment. This permits us to track a resident's ability to form a therapeutic alliance across several forms of therapy over four years of training. Since empirical evidence demonstrates that poor early alliances predict poor outcomes and early drop-outs, providing such feedback to the resident and supervisor enables more attention to be paid to ruptures in the alliance. Empathic skills, which contribute to alliance development, are assessed in the emotion-focused therapy module, which will be discussed later.

Specific therapies

Crisis intervention

Crisis intervention involves the delivery of specific integrated skills in a defined context within a supportive relationship. The primary goal of crisis intervention is to reduce acute distress, facilitate more adaptive coping skills and return the patient to a normal level of functioning. The process of therapy has been described in six stages:

1. Explicit transferring of responsibility,
2. Organize takeover of tasks,
3. Remove patient from stressful environment,
4. Lower arousal and distress,
5. Reinforce appropriate communication to encourage normal communication, and
6. Show concern, warmth and encourage hope.

(Graham and Bancroft, 2006)

In our programme, training in crisis intervention occurs in the first postgraduate year in the emergency room. Psychiatric emergency room staff first model crisis intervention, and this is then followed by the resident treating either one or two cases for a few sessions under observed supervision, or treating several patients sequentially for one session, a more realistic option in the emergency room. At present, there are no objective competency scales to assess crisis intervention skills; however, supervisors can focus on the specific skills discussed previously.

Emotion-focused therapy (supportive therapy)

Whether one is implementing pharmacotherapy, a specific psychotherapy, or a combination of both types of therapies, it is important that they be delivered in the context of a supportive relationship. Supportive interventions include active listening, attending, reflecting of thoughts and emotions, empathizing, problem-solving, giving advice, providing reassurance and making confirming comments. Although some or all of these interventions are utilized in many different forms of psychotherapy, in *supportive therapy* these interventions are considered to be the active ingredients of change, which contribute to more adaptive functioning, a decrease in symptoms, prevention of relapse, positive self-esteem, improved coping, and an increased sense of support (Barber *et al.*, 2001). Supportive therapy is indicated in many acute situations and can be combined with medication to establish a therapeutic relationship, promote alliance and increase medication compliance.

Several therapies fall under the umbrella of 'supportive therapy'. These include: client-centred therapy (Rogers, 1965), supportive–expressive therapy (Luborsky, 1984) and supportive therapy (Winston *et al.*, 2004). In our programme, residents receive training in emotion-focused therapy, an experiential therapy which incorporates client-centred and gestalt techniques (Greenberg *et al.*, 1993). This therapy was selected for training as it focuses on the core ingredients of affective exploration and empathy, and teaches residents how to attend to the patient's inner experience. This helps the resident feel comfortable with the patient's affect, and also deals with issues of depression in the context of grief, unfinished business or problematic reactions. Although certainly more sophisticated than a 'supportive therapy', it places heavy emphasis on the alliance and empathic attunement, which are essential supportive elements. The teaching of micro-counselling techniques, and moment-to-moment analysis of taped session material with feedback, are used to assist learners in the difficult task of delivering accurate empathic responses that facilitate deeper exploration (Baker and Daniels, 1989).

Competence in empathic skills is assessed using the Truax Accurate Empathy Scale (TAES). This is a nine-point anchored rating scale with good psychometric properties (Truax, 1976). Supervisors, who are uninvolved in the resident's training and blind to the session order, rate three randomly selected 10-minute segments from an early (session no 3) and late (session no 15) tape, representing early, middle and late periods in each session. These ratings are then averaged, to produce a score of one to nine for the early and late sessions. Competence is achieved with scores equal to or greater than five. Preliminary analysis with 26 residents shows significant gain in competence from early ($M = 4.38$, SD $= 2.07$) to late sessions ($M = 6.06$, SD $= 2.9$), $t(25) = 4.60$, $p = 0.0001$ (Weerasekera *et al.*, 2003). Other instruments that assess supportive therapy include the Penn Adherence Scale (Barber and Crits-Christoph, 1996), the Interpretive and Supportive Technique Scale (Ogrodniczuk and Piper, 1999), and a non-validated generic form is also available (Winston *et al.*, 2004).

Cognitive-behavioural therapy for depression

Cognitive-behavioural therapy (CBT) incorporates both cognitive and behavioural components in the conceptualization of patient problems and the delivery of treatment. The fundamental premise of CBT is that psychological distress, whether it is manifested in mood, anxiety or other problems, is a result of maladaptive thought processes, which lead to difficulties in emotions and behaviour. Treatment includes challenging these distortions in the context of a collaborative relationship and a positive therapeutic alliance.

In the CBT depression module, seminars combine an academic and practical focus with selected readings, videotapes and role-play exercises that model specific CBT skills. The final seminar teaches residents formulation and conceptualization based on the cognitive model and the interventions they have previously learned. Following the didactic component, trained supervisors utilize specific manuals to assist residents in treating depressed patients (Beck *et al.*, 1979; Greenberger and Padesky, 1995).

Competence and adherence is assessed by the primary supervisor and a second independent assessor. For this purpose, the Cognitive Therapy Scale (CTS) is used, which has been shown to have adequate psychometric properties for rating adherence and competence to CBT (Vallis *et al.*, 1986; Blackburn *et al.*, 2001). This instrument assesses general therapeutic skills, conceptualization, strategy, and techniques used in treatment. When rated by the supervisor, the CTS is completed in a formative manner, such that ratings on items are shared and discussed with the resident for the purpose of providing feedback and improving skills. In this case, no overall score is provided. Additionally, residents are required to submit tapes from an early and late session for assessment by an independent assessor who uses the CTS to derive a quantitative score. Scores of 30 to 39 (out of 66) on the CTS denote competency for novices. The information gathered from the supervisor is collated with these independent ratings to help ascertain resident competence and determine successful completion of the module. We have shown improvement in CBT skills from early to late sessions with a small group of residents and will be reporting results from a larger sample soon (Weerasekera *et al.*, 2003).

As a result of the recent RCPS guidelines, mindfulness-based cognitive therapy for depression (Segal *et al.*, 2001) has also been introduced into the programme; however, formal methods of assessing therapist competence in this area are lacking and await further study.

Cognitive-behavioural therapy for anxiety

The CBT–anxiety module focuses on training residents in the short term and on structured interventions for adults with anxiety disorders. Seminars provide an introduction to the assessment and CBT treatment for the full range of anxiety disorders. Attention is given to cognitive, exposure-based and relaxation-training strategies for each anxiety disorder. Expert supervisors use established manuals (Antony and Swinson, 2000; Barlow, 2007) to help residents deliver this brief treatment in a structured yet non-rigid manner.

Competence is assessed by the supervisor who listens to audiotapes on a weekly basis, and by an independent evaluator using the CTS (Vallis *et al.*, 1986). The assessment of resident competence in CBT for anxiety focuses more on competence in cognitive therapy, rather than in behaviour therapy. Since competence is assessed using taped sessions, it is difficult to assess therapist skill with behavioural exercises, such as in-vivo exposure sessions, which usually take place outside the office. Therapist competence in behavioural therapy is assessed informally by evaluating the resident's ability to deliver specific behavioural interventions such as obtaining baseline behaviours, creating structured activity schedules, assigning homework, reviewing homework, dealing with homework non-compliance, developing hierarchies, providing instruction in relaxation training and delivering other behavioural interventions to patients with specific psychiatric disorders.

Psychodynamic psychotherapy

Long-term psychodynamic psychotherapy is usually delivered to patients struggling with interpersonal problems, self-esteem issues, characterological problems and childhood sexual abuse issues, with a recent meta-analysis supporting its use in patients with complex problems (Leichsenring and Rabung, 2008). Although it is not the first treatment of choice in more severely ill patients with mood, anxiety and psychotic disorders, it may be an adjunctive therapy in treatment-resistant cases where more complicated issues are not treatable with medications alone or other psychological treatments.

The goal of this module is for residents to gain an understanding of the theoretical complexities and clinical techniques of psychodynamic psychotherapy through didactic lectures, small-group discussions, readings, and weekly supervision. Selected readings are assigned to assist residents in carrying out therapy with at least one case for 1–2 years of therapy. A minimum requirement, however, of completing at least 75% of one year of therapy (40 sessions) was instituted, as long as the supervisor deemed the resident to have demonstrated reasonable competence with this case. Most residents continue much longer with their patients (over two years) and carry several patients throughout their training. However, at this time formal evaluation, including the formulation submission, is carried out on only one case. Subsequent cases are evaluated by supervisors, but do not require other formal assessment procedures. Competence is assessed weekly by listening to audiotaped session material. Residents also submit a written psychodynamic formulation on their patient and their treatment process, which is assessed by the supervisor. In addition, each resident presents a formulation of a videotaped case in a seminar. At present, we do not have an objective method for assessing competence in psychodynamic skills, but are considering using measures established in the brief dynamic therapy. Skills in this module are currently assessed informally with specific attention being given to interpretive skills (especially interpretation of the transference, defences and conflicts), clarification skills, ability to show empathic attunement, provision of self-object functions and ability to attend to counter-transference. Therapist rating scales that could be utilized to assess competence are the Penn Adherence Scale (Barber and Crits-Christoph, 1996), the Interpretive and Supportive Technique Scale (Ogrodniczuk and Piper, 1999) and Luborsky's Core Conflictual Relationship Theme (CCRT) (Luborsky and Crits-Christoph, 1998). We are considering using one of these instruments.

The new guidelines also mandate that residents have introductory knowledge of brief dynamic therapy. There are several models of brief dynamic therapy (Dewan et al., 2009) and assessment of competence in this area depends on the specific model followed. Similar instruments discussed for long-term psychodynamic therapy can be used in the brief version of the model.

Family therapy

Family interventions integrated with medication or other therapies have been found to be helpful in decreasing symptoms, increasing medication compliance, and maintaining good outcomes in a variety of psychiatric disorders, such as depression, psychotic disorders, and child and adolescent disorders (MacFarlane, 2006). There are several models of family functioning and family therapy, including the McMaster model of family functioning, systems models, psychodynamic models and behavioural models (Goldenberg and Goldenberg, 2007). In our programme, the family therapy module occurs concurrently with the psychodynamic module and is integrated with the child psychiatry rotation. Objectives of this module are for residents to learn a method of family assessment, formulation and treatment through seminars and case supervision. As in other modules, videotapes are used to model specific skills and test resident knowledge base. Expert supervisors screen or view weekly videotapes of resident sessions to assess competence and provide appropriate feedback.

Competence is assessed by the supervisor and an objective evaluator, who rate early and late tapes using the Family Therapist Rating Scale (FTRS: Piercy et al., 1983). This scale assesses global therapist behaviours from diverse theoretical orientations. Five categories (with ten items in each) of therapists' behaviours are rated on a seven-point Likert scale (0–6) for a maximum score of 300. The categories include: structuring, relationship, historical, structural or process and experiential behaviours. The FTRS demonstrates good psychometric properties, with good inter-rater reliability (0.61 to 0.87) and validity, with experienced family therapists scoring higher than inexperienced therapists on each of the five subscales ($M = 162.4$ vs. $M = 93.2$, $p < 0.001$) (Piercy et al., 1983). A study correlating the five subscales with expert ratings of therapists' effectiveness, found three of the five scales to be significantly correlated (Piercy et al., 1983). A score of 100 indicates beginning skills in family therapy. Preliminary data available on a small group of residents showed gains in competence from early ($M = 121.3$, SD $= 8.08$) to late sessions ($M = 161.9$, SD $= 28.2$), $t(4) = 3.12$, $p = 0.01$ (Weerasekera et al., 2003). The small sample makes it difficult to interpret these results at this time. Hopefully, as our sample grows we can assess the utility of this scale in our programme.

Interpersonal therapy (IPT)

The fundamental assumption in IPT is that the onset, maintenance and recovery of depression are determined by four key interpersonal events: losses, role transitions, interpersonal conflicts and interpersonal deficit. Therapy focuses on integrating a medical model of depression as well as understanding and working through these key interpersonal areas (Stuart, 2003). Empirical research supports the use of IPT for depression in adults, the elderly and adolescents (Parker *et al.*, 2006).

Although the RCPS guidelines stipulate that residents must possess a working knowledge of IPT, our programme requires residents to have formal supervision to attain a beginning level of competence. Seminars expose trainees to the underlying theoretical model of IPT and videotapes that model specific techniques. Supervision is carried out with the use of well-established manuals (Weissman *et al.*, 2000) by supervisors who have received formal training in this area. To ensure adherence to IPT early in supervision, the supervisor rates an early tape using a therapy strategy rating form (TSRF; Weissman, personal communication), and provides appropriate feedback to the resident. Competency assessment involves obtaining objective ratings on the TSRF and a process rating form (PRF; Weissman, personal communication), of early (session no 3) and late (session no 12) tapes. The TSRF assesses IPT-specific interventions as well as non-specific interventions associated with a positive therapeutic alliance. The PRF is a measure of the application of IPT techniques. Overall competence is determined for both the TSRF and PRF by a total mean score of four or less on a seven-point qualitative scale where one is excellent and seven is poor. The TSRF inter-rater reliability is high with a Pearson $r = 0.88$ ($p < 0.001$), and a score of four or less is deemed to indicate therapist competence in conducting IPT (O'Malley *et al.*, 1988). Preliminary results with a small group of residents showed competence in IPT after training (Weerasekera *et al.*, 2003).

Group therapy

Group therapy can be delivered to a wide range of patients presenting with multiple disorders and several problems across the lifespan with much fewer resources than individual therapy. There is a significant body of research that supports the use of many group therapies in psychiatry. In our programme, residents initially participate as co-therapists, and later as sole therapists in some placements, utilizing manuals to deliver treatment. Although we do not formally assess competence with a specific instrument, supervisors assess the resident's knowledge base and delivery of therapy with specific markers. We are considering using specific instruments to assess group alliances with the therapist (Lindgren *et al.*, 2008).

Dialectical behaviour therapy

Dialectical behaviour therapy, originally developed for patients with borderline personality disorder, integrates features of cognitive therapy, behaviour therapy and mindfulness to promote emotional regulation, a decrease in parasuicidal behaviour and an increase in adaptive functioning (Linehan, 1993). Empirical research supports the use of DBT in patients with BPD, and in other populations

(Lynch *et al.*, 2007). In our programme, didactic seminars present the resident with basic theoretical concepts of DBT, clinical applications and the empirical literature. Residents then go on to participate as a co-therapist in a DBT group. Specific therapist skills that are assessed by the supervisor include: developing rapport and alliance, delivery of DBT, such as describing the model, psycho-education regarding the disorder, assigning homework, reviewing homework, dealing with disruptive patients in groups that challenge group dynamics, dealing with para-suicidal behaviour, non-compliance and other issues. Therapist competence is not formally assessed, although we are investigating the DBT Expert Rating scale developed by Linehan and colleagues to assess therapist competence (Linehan, private communication).

Motivational interviewing

Motivational interviewing (MI) is a specific interviewing technique aimed at assessing a patient's readiness to change to engage in treatment (Miller and Rollnick, 2002). In our programme, residents receive six weeks of training in motivational interviewing in an experiential workshop setting. After receiving the basic theoretical background, residents carry out role plays with feedback and practise MI skills. At present MI skills are assessed informally with the Motivational Interviewing Skills Code (MISC) (Miller *et al.*, 2003; Moyers *et al.*, 2003). We hope to use this instrument in a more objective fashion in the future.

Conclusion

Assessing competence in psychotherapy is a difficult and complex task. Supervisor evaluations and therapist rating scales by themselves do not provide all the answers. A skilful therapist must not only deliver the active ingredients dictated by manuals, but also form effective alliances and tailor treatments to deal with unique patient characteristics. To assist educators with the daunting task of assessment of competence, this chapter presents a competency-based psychotherapy programme that can be used as a template, in that it is portable and has already been adopted at other institutions with minor modifications. However, many issues need to be considered before adopting such a programme. Departmental support is essential to ensure that competence assessment is *mandatory*. Minimally, funding is needed for a psychotherapy coordinator (two days a week) and an administrative assistant (two days a week). Full-time medical faculty are funded through the department compensation plan. Non-MD full-time faculty receive salaries from their clinical placements, while part-time faculty earn their department appointments through providing 100 hours per year of teaching time in any programme. Where resources are poor, supervision occurs in groups, which has turned out to be a good learning experience for the residents.

Despite this support and infrastructure, considerable time and energy is required to maintain such a programme. Obtaining adherence to utilization of tapes in sessions, and submission of tapes and other evaluation material is difficult. This was especially problematic in the early phases of the programme, as philosophical differences concerning psychotherapy training and assessment had to be resolved. Recruitment and retention of skilled supervisors is also a problem. To deal with this our faculty development programme promotes in-house training and minimizes costs.

The major limitation of the programme is that with a shift to broad-based training, less emphasis has been given to one type of therapy, thereby sacrificing proficiency in any one form. Proficiency in psychotherapy, however, takes years of practice over time. Our programme has focused on establishing an adequate level of competence first, with the hope that subsequent experience will direct the resident towards specialization and later proficiency. It is also important to mention that the competency data presented in this paper were based on a 'within-subjects' design, which does not take into account improvements in general skills that develop over time. As this programme continues to develop and grow, we hope to put greater emphasis on our evaluative methods.

REFERENCES

ACGME (Accreditation Council for Graduate Medical Education) (2007). *ACGME Program Requirements for Graduate Medical Education in Psychiatry.* http://www.acgme.org/acWebsite/downloads/RRC_progReq/400_psychiatry_07012007_u04122008.pdf.

Ackerman, S. J. and Hilsenroth, M. J. (2003). A review of therapist characteristics and techniques positively impacting the therapeutic alliance. *Clinical Psychology Review,* **23,** 1–33.

Antony, M. M. and Swinson, R. P. (2000). *Phobic Disorders and Panic in Adults: A Guide to Assessment and Treatment.* Washington: American Psychological Association.

Baker, S. D. and Daniels, T. G. (1989). Integrating research on the microcounseling program: a meta-analysis. *Journal of Counseling Psychology,* **36,** 213–222.

Barber, J. P. and Crits-Christoph, P. (1996). Development of a therapist adherence/competence rating scale for supportive-expressive dynamic psychotherapy: a preliminary report, *Psychotherapy Research,* **6**(2), 81–94.

Barber, J. P., Stratt, R., Halperin, G. and Connolly, M. B. (2001). Supportive techniques: are they found in different therapies? *Journal of Psychotherapy Practice and Research,* **10**(3), 165–172.

Barlow, D. H. (ed.) (2007). *Clinical Handbook of Psychological Disorders: A Step-By-Step Treatment Manual,* 4th edn. New York: Guilford Press.

Beck, A. T., Rush, A. J., Shaw, B. F. and Emery, G. (1979). *Cognitive Therapy of Depression.* New York: Guilford Press.

Bienenfeld, D., Klykylo, W. and Lehrer, D. (2003). Closing the loop: assessing the effectiveness of psychiatric competency measures. *Academic Psychiatry,* **27**(3), 131–135.

Binks, C. A., Fenton, M., McCarthy, L. *et al.* (2006). Psychological therapies for people with borderline personality disorder. *Cochrane Database of Systematic Reviews,* **1.**

Blackburn, I. M., James, I. A., Milne, D. L. *et al.* (2001). The revised cognitive therapy scale (CTS-R): psychometric properties. *Behavioural and Cognitive Psychotherapy*, **29**, 431–446.

Bordin, E. S. (1979). The generalizability of psychoanalytic concept of the working alliance. *Psychotherapy: Theory, Research & Practice*, **16**(3), 252–260.

Burlingame, G. M., Fuhriman, A. and Mosier, J. (2003). The differential effectiveness of group psychotherapy: A meta-analytic perspective. *Group Dynamics: Theory, Research, and Practice*, **7**(1), 3–12.

Butler, A. C., Chapman, J. E., Forman, E. M. and Beck, A. T. (2006). The empirical status of cognitive-behavioral therapy: a review of meta-analyses. *Clinical Psychology Review*, **26**, 17–31.

Chevron, E. S., Bruce, M. S. and Rounsaville, J. (1983). Evaluating the clinical skills of psychotherapists. *Archives of General Psychiatry*, **40**, 1129–1132.

Cuijpers, P., van Straten, A., Andersson, G. and van Oppen, P. (2008). Psychotherapy for depression in adults: a meta-analysis of comparative outcome studies. *Journal of Consulting and Clinical Psychology*, **76**(6), 909–922.

de Mello, M. F., de Jesus Mari, J., Bacaltchuk, J., Verdeli, H. and Neugebauer, R. (2005). A systematic review of research findings on the efficacy of interpersonal therapy for depressive disorders. *European Archives of Psychiatry and Clinical Neuroscience*, **255**, 75–82.

Dewan, M., Weerasekera, P. and Stormon, L. (2009). Techniques of brief psychodynamic psychotherapy. In *Textbook of Psychotherapeutic Treatments*, ed. G. O. Gabbard, 1st edn. Washington: American Psychiatric Publishing.

Ellison, J. A., Greenberg, L. S., Goldman, R. N. and Angus, L. (2009). Maintenance of gains following experiential therapies for depression. *Journal of Consulting and Clinical Psychology*, **77**(1), 103–112.

Goldenberg, I. and Goldenberg, H. (2007). *Family Therapy: An Overview*, 7th edn. Belmont CA,: Brooks Cole.

Graham, C. and Bancroft, J. (2006). Crisis intervention. In *An Introduction to the Psychotherapies*, ed. S. Bloch, 4th edn. Oxford: Oxford University Press, pp. 197–214.

Greenberg, L. S., Rice, L. N. and Elliott, R. (1993). *Facilitating Emotional Change*. New York: Guilford Press.

Greenberger, D. and Padesky, C. A. (1995). *Mind Over Mood*, New York: Guilford Press.

Henry, W. P., Strupp, H. H., Butler, S. F., Schacht, T. E. and Binder, J. L. (1993). Effects of training in time-limited dynamic psychotherapy: changes in therapist behavior. *Journal of Consulting and Clinical Psychology*, **61**(3), 434–440.

Hettema, J., Steele, J. and Miller, W. R. (2005). Motivational interviewing. *Annual Review of Clinical Psychology*, **1**, 91–111.

Horvath, A. O. (2001). The alliance. *Psychotherapy*, **38**(4), 365–372.

Horvath, A. O. and Greenberg, L. S. (1994). *The Working Alliance: Theory, Research, and Practice*. New York: Wiley.

Leichsenring, F. and Rabung, S. (2008). Effectiveness of long-term psychodynamic psychotherapy: a meta-analysis. *JAMA*, **300**(13), 1551–1565.

Lindgren, A., Barber, J. P. and Sandahl, C. (2008). Alliance to the group-as-a-whole as a predictor of outcome in psychodynamic group therapy. *International Journal of Group Psychotherapy*, **58**(2), 163–184.

Linehan, M. (1993). *Skills Training Manual for Treating Borderline Personality Disorder*. New York: Guilford Press.

Luborsky, L. (1984). *Principles of Psychoanalytic Psychotherapy: A Manual for Supportive-Expressive Treatment*. New York: Basic Books.

Luborsky, L. and Crits-Christoph, P. (1998). *Understanding Transference: The Core Conflictual Relationship Theme Method*, 2nd edn. Washington: American Psychological Association.

Lynch, T. R., Trost, W. T., Salsman, N. and Linehan, M. M. (2007). Dialectical behavior therapy for borderline personality disorder. *Annual Review of Clinical Psychology*, **3**, 181–205.

MacFarlane, M. M. (2006). Special issue on family therapy and mental health. *Journal of Family Psychotherapy*, **17**(3–4), 1–6.

Miller, W. R. and Rollnick, S. (2002). *Motivational Interviewing: Preparing People for Change*, 2nd edn, New York: Guilford Press.

Miller, W. R., Moyers, T. B., Ernst, D. and Amrhein, P. (2003). *Manual for the Motivational Interviewing Skill Code (MISC)*. http://motivationalinterview.org/training/MISC2.pdf.

Moyers, T., Martin, T., Catley, D., Harris, K. and Ahluwalia, J. (2003). Assessing the integrity of motivational interviewing interventions: reliability of the motivational interviewing skills code. *Behavioural and Cognitive Psychotherapy*, **31**(2), 177–184.

Ogrodniczuk, J. S. and Piper, W. E. (1999). Measuring therapist technique in psychodynamic psychotherapies: development and use of a new scale. *Journal of Psychotherapy Practice and Research*, **8**(2), 142–154.

O'Malley, S. S., Foley, S. H., Rounsaville, B. J. *et al.* (1988). Therapist competence and patient outcome in interpersonal psychotherapy of depression. *Journal of Consulting and Clinical Psychology*, **56**(4), 496–501.

Parker, G., Parker, I., Brotchie, H. and Stuart, S. (2006). Interpersonal psychotherapy for depression? The need to define its ecological niche. *Journal of Affective Disorders*, **95**, 1–11.

Piercy, F. P., Laird, R. A. and Mohammed, A. (1983). A family therapist rating scale. *Journal of Marital and Family Therapy*, **9**(1), 49–59.

RCP (Royal College of Psychiatrists) (2009). *Specialist Module in Psychotherapy*. https://www.rcpsych.ac.uk/PDF/Psychotherapy_Feb09.pdf.

RCPSC (Royal College of Physicians and Surgeons of Canada) (2007). *Objectives of Training in Psychiatry*. http://rcpsc.medical.org/residency/certification/objectives/psychiatry_e.pdf.

Rogers, C. C. (1965). *Client-Centered Therapy: Its Current Practice, Implications, and Theory*. Boston: Houghton Mifflin Company.

Rowe, C. E. and MacIsaac, D. S. (1991). *Empathic Attunement: The Technique of Psychoanalytic Self-Psychology*, Northvale NJ: Jason Aronson Inc.

Segal, Z. V., Williams, J. M. G. and Teasdale, J. D. (2001). *Mindfulness-Based Cognitive Therapy for Depression: A New Approach to Preventing Relapse*, 1st edn. New York: Guilford Press.

Shadish, W. R. and Baldwin, S. A. (2003). Meta-analysis of MFT interventions. *Journal of Marital and Family Therapy*, **29**(4), 547–570.

Simmons, J., Roberge, L., Kendrick, S. B. and Richards, B. (1995). The interpersonal relationship in clinical practice: the Barrett-Lennard Relationship Inventory as an assessment instrument. *Evaluation and the Health Professions*, **18**(1), 103–112.

Stuart, S. (2003). *Interpersonal Psychotherapy*. Oxford: Oxford University Press.

Truax, C. B. (1976). A scale for the rating of accurate empathy. In *The Therapeutic Relationship and Its Impact: A Study of Psychotherapy with Schizophrenics*, ed. C. Rogers. Westport: Greenwood Press, pp. 555–568.

Vallis, T. M., Shaw, B. F. and Dobson, K. S. (1986). The cognitive therapy scale: psychometric properties. *Journal of Consulting and Clinical Psychology*, **54**(3), 381–385.

Waltz, J., Addis, M., Koerner, K. and Jacobson, N. (1993). Testing the integrity of a psychotherapy protocol assessment of adherence and competence. *Journal of Consulting and Clinical Psychology*, **61**, 620–630.

Weerasekera, P. (1997). Postgraduate psychotherapy training: incorporating findings from the empirical literature into curriculum development. *Academic Psychiatry*, **21**(3), 122–132.

Weerasekera, P. and Hnatko, G. S. (2009). Psychotherapies. In *Approaches to Postgraduate Education in Psychiatry in Canada: What Educators and Residents Need to Know*, ed. J. S. Leverette, G. S. Hnatko and E. Persad. Ottawa: Canadian Psychiatry Association Press.

Weerasekera, P., Antony, M. M., Bellissimo, A. *et al.* (2003). Competency assessment in the McMaster psychotherapy program. *Academic Psychiatry*, **27**(3), 166–173.

Weiss, K. A., Smith, T. E., Hull, J. W., Piper, A. C. and Huppert, J. D. (2002). Predictors of risk of nonadherence in outpatients with schizophrenia and other psychotic disorders. *Schizophrenia Bulletin*, **28**(2), 341–349.

Weissman, M. M., Markowitz, J. C. and Klerman, G. L. (2000). *Comprehensive Guide to Interpersonal Psychotherapy*. New York: Basic Books.

Winston, A., Rosenthal, R. N. and Pinkser, H. (2004). *Introduction to Supportive Psychotherapy*. Washington: American Psychiatric Publishing.

Yager, J. and Bienenfeld, D. (2003). How competent are we to assess psychotherapeutic competence in psychiatric residents? *Academic Psychiatry*, **27**(3), 174–181.

12

Assessments and their utility: looking to the future

Valerie Wass

Editors' introduction

Previous chapters in this book have discussed the current state of the art within assessments in postgraduate medical and, more specifically, psychiatric training. Training and assessment developments and challenges from countries around the world have also been outlined. In this final chapter, Valerie Wass, herself a leading figure in international medical education, outlines some of the conceptual and pragmatic debates that are currently occurring within the medical education world. These debates and their outcome are likely to define the next decade of postgraduate psychiatric assessments. It is argued that at the current stage of technical and educational development, although workplace-based assessments may have high authenticity and validity, on their own they may not be sufficient to enable high-stake decision-making. The balance between reliability and validity is crucial for the overall utility of the assessment programme and a combination of workplace-based assessments and standardized examinations is required for a reliable and valid assessment process. Wass also cautions against the tick-box culture that can be promoted by competency-based assessments and asserts that excellence rather than competence should be the goal of all educational programmes. It is recommended that assessment processes take into account the cognitive evolution of trainees as they progress from novicehood to expertise. Finally, formative and summative components of an assessment process must be adequately balanced with the ultimate aim of achieving maximum educational impact.

Introduction

Most of the change we think we see in life is due to truths being in and out of favour. (Robert Frost)

Workplace-Based Assessments in Psychiatric Training, ed. Dinesh Bhugra and Amit Malik.
Published by Cambridge University Press. © Cambridge University Press 2011.

Over the past 40 years we have seen significant changes in assessment. The balance first swung, originally in North America, to a culture where reliability and defensibility began to dominate. The need to assess clinical competence in a legally defensible manner was perceived to be of paramount performance. Clinical long and short case studies were abandoned because of a lack of reliability. This change occurred in the face of surprisingly little published data on their psychometric performance (van der Vleuten, 1996a). Knowledge tests came to the fore. There was a strong move to the multiple-choice test format, which enabled wide testing across a range of contexts, thus ensuring that context specificity and reliability were fully addressed. This was an important move. Professionals do not perform consistently across tasks set in different contexts. The change acknowledged the need to sample widely across a clinician's expertise. The crucial importance of context specificity, when assessing clinical competency, is perhaps the most important evidence-based assessment truth. It cannot be ignored. Objective structured examinations followed (Harden and Gleeson, 1979) as the more traditional formats were abandoned. For those of us involved in the change to these more structured objective tests, concerns for loss of validity were very much apparent (Talbot, 2004). Yet most now regard these formats as fairer. They recognize the risk of using a limited number of unstructured cases if reliability is to be achieved in high-stake testing. We have learnt from this change.

Loss of validity, though, remained an important concern. Subsequently evidence began to emerge that the assessment method itself was, in actuality, not the key to reliability (van der Vleuten and Schuwirth, 2005). The length and breadth of sampling is the more decisive factor. As long as the method sampled a sufficient range of case material and addressed context specificity, traditional tools held their value. Ten long case studies (Wass *et al.*, 2001) or three hours of oral examinations (Wass *et al.*, 2003) were potentially as reliable as an OSCE. The pendulum swung back towards validity. A move to re-develop more traditional assessment tools for the workplace was founded. The mini-CEX, for example, is essentially a modification of the long case assessment and the case-based discussion of an oral examination. As illustrated in the previous chapters, assessment practice became much more inventive as modifications of more traditional approaches came back into favour.

Few would argue that we have as yet achieved a gold standard or, indeed, ever will. There is no ideal assessment. Van der Vleuten's utility equation, as outlined in Chapter 1, emphasizes the need to balance various facets of assessment according to the purpose of the test (van der Vleuten, 1996b):

$$\text{Utility} = \text{Reliability} \times \text{Validity} \times \text{Feasibility} \times \text{Acceptability}$$
$$\times \text{Educational impact.}$$

Workplace-based assessment is no exception. It is unlikely to prove a Utopia and free us from all other approaches to clinical competency testing. In looking to the future, there are practical and conceptual challenges still to be addressed. The need to balance assessment programmes according to their purpose and potential is of paramount importance. The challenges lie in producing workplace-based assessments which:

1. Weigh reliability against validity;
2. Strive to achieve excellence and not just competence;
3. Acknowledge the progression from novice to an expert;
4. Balance formative and summative assessment to achieve educational impact.

Weighing validity against reliability

Everything that can be counted does not necessarily count; everything that counts cannot necessarily be counted. (Albert Einstein)

Einstein's words reflect the conundrum we face when designing workplace-based assessment programmes. Many believe that multiple-choice test papers and objective structured examinations fail to 'count' the competencies we aim to 'count'. Yet they are of proven reliability. Will the new workplace-based methodology prove robust enough to replace these formats and achieve the validity needed to 'count' such aspects as professional behaviour? This may be too aspirational.

To date it remains doubtful that workplace-based assessment can ever achieve the degree of reliability required to make high-stake decisions on progression legally defensible. The format relies heavily on a framework that guarantees adequate coverage of the curriculum and tests trainees across a range of clinical problems set in different contexts. We are all human and, albeit if unconsciously, tend to focus on our 'wants' rather than our 'needs'. Careful educational supervision and direction by appropriately trained assessors is essential to support effective testing across the curriculum. As yet we lack evidence on exactly how many of the different available tools are needed and how these should be combined to maximize reliability. We work in environments where time is at a premium and providing adequate appropriately trained assessors may not prove feasible.

The assessment of the UK Foundation programme (http://www.foundationprogramme.nhs.uk/pages/home), for the initial two years post graduation, is entirely based on formative workplace-based methodology. Acknowledging that content specificity and assessor inconsistency represent the greatest threats to reliability, trainees are asked to use different clinical problems and assessors for each assessment. The results are encouraging (Davies et al., 2009). They suggest that confidence limits can be set to identify trainees who are performing satisfactorily. At the same time, the methodology has the potential to highlight those needing more extensive supervision and assessment. Confidence limits for the different tools can be measured. We still lack psychometric data to explore the overall combined reliability of the programme. In contrast with standardized examinations, each trainee has undertaken a completely unique assessment. Faced with current evidence, we can only conclude that workplace-based assessment offers a level of reliability appropriate to moderate-stake assessments. This can inform progression through training programmes but still lacks the robustness required of high-stake licensing tests.

Does workplace-based assessment necessarily 'count' what we aim to 'count'? Validity as a conceptual concept is challenging to measure (Downing, 2003). Correlations between the results from different workplace tools have been calculated to explore hypotheses based on the intended focus of assessment and hence their validity. For example, multi-source feedback, which assesses humanistic aspects of performance, would be expected to show a relatively low correlation with direct observation of procedures, which focuses on technical expertise. There is a growing body of evidence supporting the validity of the most frequently used tools, such as the mini-CEX and case-based discussion. Meaningful correlations are seen both between individual workplace-based tools and against performance on more traditional examinations, such as written tests and orals (Norcini and Burch, 2007). At the same time, there is some confirmatory data suggesting that trainees' scores do improve over time (Davies *et al.*, 2009). This evidence is reassuring in terms of validating the tools.

As we look to the future there may also be a need to revisit our conceptual thinking. Although workplace-based assessment observes performance in the workplace, if we refer back to Miller's pyramid (see Chapter 1), this arguably risks measuring 'shows how' rather than 'does.' The model implicitly assumes that competence, demonstrated under controlled conditions set by the assessment tool, predicts practice in the real world. Yet the very act of observing a system, in this case the workplace, will in itself affect that system. A key principle, the Hawthorne effect, almost certainly comes into play. This is essentially an observer effect; efficiency and performance can change simply as a result of workers being observed. There is no guarantee that the improvement, which observation appears to catalyze, will be maintained in the long term. This can affect the validity of tests. They assure competency at a fixed point in time. We lack evidence that this is either maintained over time or, indeed, accurately reflects the trainee's unobserved behaviour.

Several studies have shown differences between doctors' performance in controlled assessments and the reality of their actual practice (Rethans *et al.* 1991; Southgate *et al.*, 2001). Other influences, related both to the individual (stress, health) and systems (conditions of practice), can impact significantly on performance. Competence ('shows how') sheds light on performance but does not fully illuminate it. There has been a reconsideration of Miller's model, stimulated by a belief that it lacks the flexibility to reflect the actuality of unobserved workplace performance. Rethans *et al.* (2002) suggest inverting the pyramid to place greater weight on performance. They argue that this modification highlights additional individual- and system-related influences. Their paper offers a useful reflection of the challenges faced when moving assessment from the relatively controlled environment of the examination hall to the reality of postgraduate training in the workplace. As we move forward, new approaches to conceptual ideology should be encouraged.

We need more evidence. Research into the validity and reliability of workplace methodologies is essential. New developments must be robustly constructed and analyzed to enhance our understanding of how appropriate frameworks for assessment can be established, weighing purpose with required outcomes. At this point in time, the emerging evidence suggests that we are on the right track. Workplace-based assessment does have a place but is not reliable enough to substitute for more traditional summative assessments of learning. The authenticity and validity of workplace assessment can supplement the more reliable, but typically less valid, traditional examinations. It weighs more heavily on the side of validity than reliability and cannot stand alone. Workplace-based programmes and standardized assessments need to be combined to achieve valid and reliable licensing processes.

Striving to achieve excellence and not just competence

All labour that uplifts humanity has dignity and importance and should be undertaken with painstaking excellence. (Martin Luther King, Jr)

A frequently voiced concern is that workplace-based assessment encourages a tick-box culture (PMETB, 2010). This potential limitation cannot be ignored. Once trainees have completed an assessment, it remains imperative that they continue to practise and develop professionally. In both undergraduate and postgraduate education, a genuine risk is emerging that, once the box is ticked, trainees consider themselves to be fully competent to carry out the task. They then fail to continue to practise; an essential component of skills development. This concern was strongly expressed by the working party convened by the Royal College of Physicians in the UK (RCP, 2005) to address professionalism in the twenty-first century. To quote the report:

Competence means the ability or capacity to do something. We wanted to set a higher standard than mere capability. Instead, excellence stresses the possession of abilities to an eminent or meritorious degree. A good doctor should not only have a skill. He or she should be able to demonstrate the exercise of that skill in an especially worthwhile way, a concept better served, we believe, by the idea of working towards excellence. (RCP, 2005)

The challenge for the development of workplace-based assessment remains the need to design programmes that encourage and reward excellence and not just competence.

Attempts have been made to define stages of competence that embrace the need for continuing professional development (Weigel *et al.*, 2007). Yet arguably the tools being developed do encourage a tick-box culture. They falsely assure trainees that they are fully competent on the task being assessed. This is reinforced by the relatively high scores trainees receive in the first half of the two-year UK Foundation programme (Davies *et al.*, 2009). If we are to encourage progression,

WPBA requires a radical change in assessment culture. This applies equally to trainees and assessors.

Consider the trainees' perspective. Doctors are selected through a process which requires top levels of academic achievement. They tend to be competitive and set high expectations of themselves. Low scores risk being viewed as 'failure' by trainees. They have difficulty recognizing that this form of assessment is designed to offer learning opportunities for personal development and improvement. Instead, assessment is deferred until they can foresee a good score. As a result, the opportunity to receive feedback and learn is lost in order to avoid a low mark. In the analysis of the UK Foundation programme, 40% of trainees submitted their assessments in the last four weeks (Davies *et al.*, 2009). We need to emphasize to both trainees and assessors that less than perfect scores early in training should be the norm and will be viewed positively. Through informed feedback and further practice, progressive improvement is to be expected. Observing an incremental change in scores is essential and should be rewarded.

Assessors come from a similar culture. They tend to award high marks avoiding the lower range of scores (Davies *et al.*, 2009). It is important that we understand why. In the one-to-one feedback process, a high mark may be viewed as encouraging. Alternatively, this may reflect inadequate assessor training. As we proceed, we need to know much more about how assessors formulate their judgements and ensure that they are appropriately trained.

Following a target-driven 'ticking-boxes' approach with the aim of achieving a high score defeats the purpose of workplace-based assessment. It fails in its aspiration to encourage reflection and development, monitor progress and guide learning. Workplace-based assessment should be recognized as a series of essential educational events along a learning trajectory. The culture, both for trainees and assessors, needs to move away from regarding the assessment tools as end points, in the way that traditional formal examinations are viewed. Demonstration of a progressive increase in levels of achievement is to be encouraged. This is a radical change in culture where high scores lose value and the reward lies in formulating ways of raising performance with an explicit goal of excellence.

Acknowledging the progression from novice to expert

We do not receive wisdom. We must discover it for ourselves after experience which no-one else can have for us and from which no-one can spare us. (Marcel Proust)

As highlighted, clinical competence is a complex construct embracing the need to integrate cognitive, psychomotor and affective skills. The pathway for learning diagnostic reasoning is, to a significant extent, dependent and resultant on clinical experience. The move from a novice to an expert is a complex cognitive process (Schmidt and Norman, 2007). The gradual assimilation of knowledge and skills is resultant on personal experience. Trainees progressively 'encapsulate' knowledge into diagnostics labels and then move into automatic patterns of disease recognition known as 'illness scripts'. These are more narrative than factual, derive from everyday clinical practice, and almost completely 'bypass' the original building blocks with which a novice works. They are cognitive entities containing relatively little basic knowledge and are scaffolded from direct patient encounters; a product of growing clinical experience. Similarly the steps required of procedural skills become increasingly assimilated with practice into an automated integrated performance. Not surprisingly, 'illness scripts' can be very individual as clinical experience is so varied. As Eraut (1994) points out:

'Expert' performance is often tacit; identifying aspects of different disciplinary practices is in itself a significant task.

This 'mismatch' between the reasoning processes of a novice and those of an expert explains some of the dilemmas faced when developing workplace-based assessment.

If we expect our future clinicians to be excellent, we must begin to test across the education continuum at increasingly higher skill levels or, perhaps more importantly, use assessment to drive professional development. Assessment methods must be tailored to accommodate shifts in reasoning, which develop implicitly with experience. Programmes must be formulated accordingly. They should respect both the education continuum and the progressive integration of knowledge with psychomotor and affective skills. An emerging pitfall, when designing workplace-based assessment, lies in a failure to refer back to prior learning and build on this to raise the challenge. A spiral curriculum is important (Harden, 1999). Yet we tend to overlook and lose the necessary continuum both across undergraduate into postgraduate and across core into specialist training transitions. It is important to identify a trainee's position on the novice-to-expert pathway and encourage a higher level of reasoning or clinical performance. Designing assessments to achieve this can be challenging. It is essential to ask the question repeatedly: 'Is this assessment appropriate to the cognitive level of the trainees as they progress towards clinical expertise?' An explicit pathway of progression may in itself aid the development of a culture that supports professional development across transitions within training programmes.

There are other important pitfalls, which need to be addressed. We know that clinicians tend to mark a trainees' performance more reliably using a global rather than check-list rating (Regehr et al., 1998). Our understanding of the cognitive pathways involved in the encapsulation of knowledge and formation of illness scripts supports this observation. An assessor automatically marks capability against an internalized standard, which has become implicit over time. One can argue that this has a powerful impact on assessment in the workplace in two ways.

Clinicians internalize different standards and approaches to practice in individual ways, nurtured by their experiences. Extensive assessor training is required to ensure consistency of judgement between physicians. Some may place greater weight on certain aspects of performance than others do. For some, an omission by a trainee may affect their interpretation more profoundly if, for example, they have had a difficult experience in that particular area. Both trainers and assessors must have a good understanding of the criteria against which judgements are being made. They need to be able to compromise if the agreed standard does not necessarily match their own. We face an uncomfortable truth. There is a need to *select* as well as *train* assessors (Wakeford *et al.*, 1995). Not everyone has the necessary skills. A prime example occurs if an assessor has different standards from those required and is unprepared to change. In the workplace this is clearly more difficult to enforce. A selection and training process can be more easily established and implemented for a panel of assessors to support an examination. Ensuring an adequate level of inter-assessor reliability in the workplace is challenging. This inevitably impacts on overall reliability, confining it to a level of moderate- rather than high-stake assessment requirements. Whether these practicalities can ever be overcome remains to be seen.

Clinicians need to be clear at what point on the novice-to-expert pathway they are formulating their judgements. This is emerging as another important aspect of assessor training. In a two-year training programme, for example, the intention should be to judge the trainee against the exit standard. This ensures that trainees have goals for progressive improvement across the course. Yet a tendency is emerging for some assessors to judge performance against where they expect the trainee to be at that point in time, rather than at the end of the two years. This may partly explain the high ratings given early in the course. It may reflect that assessors find this standard easier to internalize. Alternatively, it avoids giving and justifying to the trainee a low rating, which some may find difficult. Once again, more research is required to understand this process.

Finally, the assessor's position on the novice-to-expert pathway it is proving to be important. Expert assessors appear to assess more accurately than junior members of the team. The latter tend to overestimate competency. Emerging evidence (Wilkinson *et al.*, 2008) suggests, not surprisingly, that the more senior expert staff are more objective judges. They give lower, but more accurate, ratings than less senior members of the team. Yet, given the pressure on senior staff in the workplace, the risk is that assessments are delegated to less experienced staff who have not yet internalized the required standard or been trained in the process.

Workplace-based assessment assesses across a novice-to-expert developmental process in contrast with the traditional end point. This appears to have intrinsic difficulties. We need more research to understand these. Making judgements can be facilitated if agreed behavioural word descriptors are available on which to anchor them. These descriptors need to be transparent to both trainees and assessors, clearly outlining the level of performance required. There is emerging evidence that this is more effective than allocating a score (PMETB, 2010). Ensuring that these descriptors anchor the performance at the appropriate point in the novice-to-expert progression is of paramount importance.

Balancing formative and summative assessment to achieve educational impact

The task of the modern educator is not to cut down jungles, but to irrigate deserts. (C. S. Lewis)

Arguably the most important facet of the utility equation is that it places emphasis on harnessing assessment to ensure educational impact. This is of utmost importance. Education is implicit to the formative philosophy of workplace assessment, which was formulated as a means of progressively 'irrigating' the trainee's professional development. This originated as a strong initiative to replace summative examinations with more formative assessment programmes, which reflect the socio-cultural milieu of the curriculum (van der Vleuten and Schuwirth, 2005). Educational supervision and constructive advice for personal development is the prime aim. The validity of judgements made by tutors, and the formative potential of their feedback, takes precedence. Setting objectives for improvement must be based on robust, valid critiques of performance. There is compelling evidence that giving formative feedback to learners, while assessing them in the workplace, can improve achievement (Norcini and Burch, 2007).

Yet in reality summative judgements are almost invariably also required. A decision-making function is invariably placed on the process. Trainees have to complete workplace-based assessments successfully to inform progression decisions even if the final judgement includes a standardized examination. The aim of highlighting and supporting struggling trainees requires precise reliable records. These are essential to ensure effective feedback and ultimately defend challenge from the trainee if extra training or, rarely, exclusion from the programme results. The defensibility required of the judgements places a significant weight on their reliability. Tutors are being asked to collaborate formatively with trainees and give regular feedback on performance. As discussed, this socio-cultural approach creates a tension for tutors within the pressures of their working day. At the same time, they may be asked to make summative judgements on the trainee's competence to practise. These roles entail very different power relations, which can be difficult to enact side by side; a dilemma that cannot be ignored. There has, to date, been very little exploration in the literature on how assessments can be combined (if indeed they can) to balance formative and summative purposes within the same process. We need to improve our understanding on how to achieve this and support assessors in this difficult feedback role, which can embrace both formative and summative tasks. As discussed, removing scores from the process and focusing assessment on word descriptors is now recommended (PMETB, 2010). This enables both the facets of the competency being assessed and the level of achievement required to be verbally expressed. In theory, the word picture created should better support formative feedback. Work in the education sector confirms this. Learning outcomes appear to be optimum when verbal feedback is given alone without a concomitant score. We need to understand more on the impact of feedback on trainee learning behaviour and performance. To date, there is very little information about the strategic use of formative assessment in the workplace context to drive the learning of medical trainees. The need for such data is apparent. Not only do we need to determine the impact of feedback on learning behaviour, we also need to understand how sustainable benefits in workplace-based performance can be achieved through successful formative assessment strategies.

Training to give feedback in the workplace is essential yet difficult to achieve and not always feasible. Faculty development is critical to the quality and effectiveness of formative assessment. Well-established educational principles apply. Efficacy of feedback is enhanced if it is consistent with the needs of the learner, focuses on important aspects of the performance in the workplace, and is immediate and specific. Unfortunately, evidence to date suggests that this does not necessarily happen in practice. The assessment of directly observed performance as part of routine educational practice has been infrequent; the long case assessment, for example, was traditionally unobserved (Wass and Jolly, 2001). Evidence suggests that ensuring that trainees are observed can be an initial stumbling block; physicians may succumb to the understandable pressures of work and save time on this part of the process. We face again a need to change the culture. In addition, the quality of feedback, when given, may be poor. Inadequate or even no feedback may be offered (Norcini and Burch, 2007). Perhaps most importantly there is a need to change the response of trainees to feedback. Holmboe and colleagues (2004) in the USA demonstrated that after mini-CEX encounters only a third elicited any form of self-evaluation by the trainee and that only 8% of mini-CEX encounters were translated into a plan of action. Similar findings are emerging in the undergraduate arena. Strategies to encourage both faculty and trainees to engage in and follow the underlying philosophy of formative feedback in the workplace are critical to its future successful implementation.

Making negative judgements is culturally difficult for trainers unless support is in place for them as well as trainees. Some fear 'whistle blowing' if a trainee is struggling or significantly risks not achieving the necessary standard for completion and progression. There is an apparent tendency to avoid hard judgements in relation to the trainee's future and assume that others further down the line will make the more difficult decisions. This may reflect unfamiliarity with the system or an assessors' reluctance to be responsible for giving a trainee a poor assessment. The different power relations that challenge an assessor when asked to combine formative and summative roles come into play. It is important for assessors to recognize that their individual assessment is only part of an overall trainee profile. Failure to record and feed back areas for development is detrimental to patient safety, the trainee and the professionalism of the assessor.

To date, 'formative' and 'summative' have been used as dichotomous assessment terms. If workplace assessment is to be reliably used to inform competency decisions we need to understand more about the implications of combining these functions. Formative assessment risks being used to support and develop learners with little emphasis on psychometric principles. Psychometricians' preoccupation with reliability is viewed as the preserve of summative assessment; ensuring that pass–fail decisions are robust. As a result, feedback on performance is rarely given after summative assessment beyond a pass–fail decision. Continuing to view formative and summative assessment as separate processes is not progressive. Learners, whether they pass or fail, are entitled to expect detailed feedback on their performance. It should perhaps be argued that all assessment must be able to demonstrate reliable psychometric properties. As workplace-based assessment progresses, more attention must be paid to the development of psychometrically robust formative tools. Arguably, if the main aim is to provide feedback, then the information given must be both valid and reliable. Research is urgently needed to address this cultural change as we move away from the formative–summative dichotomy.

Conclusions

Since the seminal paper from van der Vleuten and Schuwirth (2005), progress has undoubtedly been made in developing a more formative approach to assessment in the workplace. As emphasized in the introductory chapter, any claim that WPBA is superior to, or can replace, summative examinations has not been realized. At its best, WPBA can achieve moderate reliability. The gain in validity is almost inevitably at the expense of some loss in reliability. Workplace-based assessment is still best used alongside established summative examination procedures. The main challenge lies in combining formative and summative goals.

Our aim over the next decade should be to inculcate in the working environment a more formative educational culture. The hurdles set in place by working time directives, management targets and traditional attitudes must be overcome. Arguably, the trainees themselves could lead this. However, they too face a radical change in the values they have hitherto placed on assessment. They need to switch from the competitive high-achievement goals set by examinations to a more formative culture where working with relatively low scores to set action plans in place for improvement becomes the norm. Research to improve our understanding of feedback processes from both the assessee's and assessor's perspective is essential.

Assessors need to learn to give more constructive formative feedback and trainees require support in converting feedback into learning processes. Both are crucial to ensure assessment motivates trainees to strive for excellence and, ultimately, the highest standards of patient care. The emerging concerns that we are creating a 'tick-off' competency culture must be addressed. If the new assessment culture gains sound foundations in undergraduate education and, arguably, schools, we can be optimistic that highly effective WPBA will in time gain a seamless place in postgraduate training. In the meantime careful analysis of the learning gained from, and questions raised in this book, should hopefully stimulate further research. This is essential to aid our understanding of how to manage this fundamental change.

REFERENCES

Davies, H., Archer, J., Southgate, L. and Norcini, J. J. (2009). Initial evaluation of the first year of the Foundation Assessment Programme. *Medical Education*, **43**, 74–81.

Downing, S. M. (2003). Validity: on the meaningful interpretation of assessment data. *Medical Education*, **37**, 830–837.

Eraut, M. (1994). *Developing Professional Knowledge and Competence.* London: Falmer Press.

Harden, R. M. (1999). What is a spiral curriculum? *Medical Teacher*, **21**, 141–143.

Harden, R. M. and Gleeson, F. A. (1979). Assessment of medical competence using an objective structured clinical examination (OSCE). *Journal of Medical Education*, **13**, 41–54.

Holmboe, E. S., Yepes, M., Williams, F. and Huot, S. J. (2004). Feedback and the miniclinical evaluation exercise. *Journal of General Internal Medicine*, **19**, 558–561.

Norcini, J. J. and Burch, V. (2007). Workplace-based assessment as an educational tool: AMEE Guide No. 31. *Medical Teacher*, **29**, 855–871.

PMETB (Postgraduate Medical Education Training Board) (2010). *Workplace Based Assessment: A Guide for Implementation.* General Medical Council. http://www.gmc-uk.org/Workplace_Based_Assessment.pdf_31300577.pdf.

RCP (Royal College of Physicians) UK (2005). *Doctors in Society: Medical Professionalism in a Changing World.* www.rcplondon.ac.uk/pubs/books/docinsoc.

Regehr, G., MacRae, H., Reznick, R. and Szalay, D. (1998). Comparing the psychometric properties of checklists and global rating scales for assessing performance on an OSCE-format examination. *Academic Medicine*, **73**, 993–997.

Rethans, J. J., Sturmans, F., Drop, R., van der Vleuten, C. and Hobus, P. (1991). Does competence of general practitioners predict their performance? Comparison between examination setting and actual practice. *BMJ*, **303**, 1377–1380.

Rethans, J. J., Norcini, J. J., Baron-Maldonado, M., Blackmore, D. and Jolly, B. C. (2002). The relationship between competence and performance: implications for assessing practice performance. *Medical Education*, **36**, 901–909.

Schmidt, H. G. and Norman, G. R. (2007). How expertise develops in medicine: knowledge encapsulation and illness script formation. *Medical Education*, **41**, 1133–1139.

Southgate, L., Campbell, M., Cox, J. *et al.* (2001). The General Medical Council's performance procedures: the development and implementation of tests of competence with examples from general practice. *Medical Education* **35**(suppl. 1), 20–28.

Talbot, M. (2004). Monkey see, monkey do: a critique of the competency model in graduate medical education. *Medical Education*, **38**, 587–592.

van der Vleuten, C. P. M. (1996a). Making the best of the "long case". *Lancet*, **347**, 704–705.

van der Vleuten, C. P. M. (1996b). The assessment of professional competence: developments, research and practical implications. *Advances in Health Sciences Education*, **1**, 41–67.

van der Vleuten, C. P. M. and Schuwirth, L. W. T. (2005). Assessing professional competence: from methods to programmes. *Medical Education*, **39**, 309–317.

Wakeford, R., Southgate, L. and Wass, V. (1995). Improving oral examinations: selecting, training and monitoring examiners for the MRCGP. *BMJ*, **311**, 931–935.

Wass, V. and Jolly, B. (2001). Does observation add to the validity of the long case? *Medical Education*, **35**, 729–734.

Wass, V., Jones, R. and van der Vleuten, C. P. M. (2001). Standardised or real patients to test clinical competence? The long case revisited. *Medical Education*, **35**, 321–325.

Wass, V., Wakeford, R., Neighbour, R. and van der Vleuten, C. P. M. (2003). Achieving acceptable reliability in oral examinations: an analysis of the Royal College of General Practitioner's membership examination's oral component. *Medical Education*, **37**, 126–131.

Weigel, T., Mulder, M. and Collins, K. (2007). The concept of competency in the development of vocational education and training in selected EU member states. *Journal of Vocational Education and Training*, **59**, 53–66.

Wilkinson, J., Crossley, J., Wragg, A. *et al.* (2008). Implementing workplace-based assessment across the medical specialties in the United Kingdom. *Medical Education*, **42**, 364–373.

Index